the **one-minute** meditator

the **one-minute** meditator

*relieving stress and
finding meaning in everyday life*

David Nichol, MD
and Bill Birchard

PERSEUS PUBLISHING

Cambridge, Massachusetts

A CIP record for this book is available from the Library of Congress.

The art for this book was created by Meryl Henderson.

The meditation icon was created by Sandy Overbey.

Printed in the United States of America.

Perseus Publishing is a member of the Perseus Books Group

Text design by Jeffrey P. Williams
Set in 11-point Goudy by Perseus Publishing Services

Visit us on the World Wide Web at http://www.perseuspublishing.com

Perseus Publishing books are available at special discounts for bulk purchases in the U.S. by corporations, institutions, and other organizations. For more information, please contact the Special Markets Department at HarperCollins Publishers, 10 East 53rd Street, New York, NY 10022, or call 1–212–207–7528.

First printing, March 2001
1 2 3 4 5 6 7 8 9 10—03 02 01

Contents

Preface   vii

1 The One-Minute Mind   1

2 The One-Minute Escape   31

3 The Drive for Peace   51

4 One-Minute Meditation   73

5 One-Minute Medicine   101

6 Different Strokes   127

7 The *New* One-Minute Mind   153

Further Reading   163

Preface

We invite you to become a one-minute meditator. If you accept, expect us to take you on a journey. A journey that starts as you explore how stress comes into your life. A journey that ends as you learn how to leave stress behind. As you approach your destination, you will find that your life changes. You will find more meaning.

The focus of this book is on the time span of one minute. Why? Because the quality of our lives revolves around how we feel minute to minute. Not hour to hour. Not day to day. Not year to year. Minute to minute. Within just one minute, we may experience the darkest parts of our lives. Or the brightest. In one instant, we may suffer the painful pinpricks of stress. In the next we may revel in all the fullness and mystery of life.

In the past, you may have felt you had little choice in which way your next minute would go. Your minutes may not have been your own. A swift turn of events could have filled the next minute with great satisfaction. Or could have taken from that minute all the joy of living. But the fact is, you can always take concrete steps to turn that next minute into a chance for better living.

This book shows you how. One step at a time. One meditation at a time. In each chapter, we offer three "one-minute meditations." After just the first four chapters, you will find that in using these meditations and in reading the text you've passed the four most critical milestones on your journey to reduced stress and increased well-being:

➤ *Touring your mind.* Seeing the mental traffic of the mind—along with the congestion and conflict that provoke stress and anxiety.

➤ *Viewing your escapes.* Recognizing the trial-and-error means you use to control stress—and how they don't quite work.

➤ *Seeing your potential.* Understanding that we all have within us a "drive for peace," whatever our lifestyle or beliefs.

➤ *Tapping your potential.* Learning how to build an enduring sense of contentedness using the formal skills of meditation.

This journey is a program for learning meditation on your own. Where does this program come from? From the latest thinking on how the mind works. From the latest medical research on stress and stress-reduction through meditation. From the experience of meditation teachers over the ages. And from our own experience.

We each have meditated for more than twenty-five years. After finishing months of instruction in Asia, David taught Bill in college how to sit in meditation. Since then, we both have learned from some of the world's most renowned teachers and physicians. David has devoted his life to healing minds and bodies through healthy foods, yoga, massage therapy, meditation, medications, psychotherapy, and psychoanalysis. His patients have repeatedly benefited from his teaching meditation as a new skill to make life calmer, richer, deeper.

Our combined experience convinced us that the best way to explain meditation is to focus on "the minute." This minute right now. Everyone can grasp the idea of a minute. Everyone can remember a minute. Today, everyone cares about making the best use of *every* minute—especially the challenge of spending the next one wisely. By focusing on the minute, we have reduced the concepts of meditation to something simple.

To get the most out of our book, we encourage you to get involved in it. Involved mentally as you try our meditations. Involved emotionally as you read the stories of other meditators. We've written this book in a simple, fast-paced style to make your involvement easier. We hope that our straightforward plan encourages you to put meditation to work. Not only can it reduce stress right now, it can alleviate long-term ailments like heart disease, asthma, and anxiety disorders.

You can reduce stress in ways other than by using meditation. If you've talked with your doctor, you've heard plenty about exercise, eating right, slowing down, keeping close friends, and so on. We recommend that you take this advice to heart. But note that none of these lifestyle habits—however healthy—directly address the root cause of stress: the mind. You—or you in consultation with your doctor—should consider meditation as a direct means to stop stress from spiraling out of control.

A word of caution: Often, prescription medication may be the right way to handle stress and anxiety. Ask your doctor for his or her advice. But remember that all medications have side effects, and some medications lose their effect over time. Ask your doctor about them. You may serve yourself best if you devise a stress-reduction strategy that complements your use of medication. For some people, ongoing medication is necessary. But for many, medication may be an interim aid on the path toward peace of mind.

We believe you will enjoy this book precisely because we've asked so many people to help us write it. First of all, we interviewed three dozen meditators to gather firsthand stories of people learning meditation. We chose about a dozen of them—nurse, secretary, law clerk, plant manager, student, retiree, and so on—to illustrate our points. We have changed these people's identities to protect their privacy. We asked all of them to check their stories for accuracy. We want to thank these people to no end. They make our book come alive.

We also benefited from dozens of teachers, friends, physicians, and psychologists. Many have contributed thoughts. Some have reviewed drafts. All have encouraged and inspired us. We want to say thank-you to our band of advisers: Sylvia Boorstein (author, *It's Easier Than It Looks*), Jeryn Langensand (Healthtrac), Flynn O'Malley, Ph.D. (Menninger Behavioral Health), and Marcie Parker, Ph.D. (United Healthcare).

We want to thank the physicians who reviewed the text: William H. Birchard (Sr.), M.D., and Janet Bodle, M.D. We also want to thank the following for reading early drafts of the book: Geoff Birchard, Ph.D., Jared Brown, Jean Clark, Liz Nichol, Peter Nichol, and John Riker, Ph.D.

We want to thank the pioneers and experts in this field as well. Beyond talking with many of them, we have been informed and inspired by their work over the years: Robert Aitken, Herbert Benson, M.D., Elmer Green, Ph.D., Jon Kabat-Zinn, Ph.D., Jack Kornfield, Ph.D., Anagarika

Munindra, Seung Sahn, Roger Walsh, M.D., Ph.D., and Shinzen Young.

We want to thank our editor, Marnie Cochran, and our agent, Nancy Love, for making this book possible. They embraced our ideas early. They had the faith, vision, and enthusiasm to invest in our work when our book was just a skeleton of ideas. We are forever grateful.

Finally, we want to thank our close friends and families, who have been so supportive. We dedicate the book to our parents, Bill and Millie Birchard and the late Henry and Betty Nichol. We treasure their steady support, lively interest, and unswerving examples of full living.

There is only one world,
the world pressing against you at this minute.
There is only one minute in which you are alive,
this minute here and now.
The only way to live is by accepting each minute
as an unrepeatable miracle.

—STORM JAMESON, NOVELIST, 1891–1986

the **one-minute** meditator

1

The One-Minute Mind

Don't believe everything you think.

—UNKNOWN

Five Breaths. You are about to take the first step in learning to meditate. Start by settling comfortably in your seat. Close your eyes. Slowly, deeply draw in a breath. Feel your chest rise and your belly expand. Inhale until you feel your lung tissue stretch and flood with oxygen. Now exhale slowly. Let your chest relax, your belly go limp. Then take four more breaths the same way.

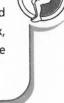

Your breathing can be ever so relaxing. Why? Because, believe it or not, your mind follows your breath. As you deliberately savor the cool air flowing in, and feel the warm air coursing out, you slow the flow of your thoughts and emotions. As you slow your breath, you soothe your mind. As an experiment, try the reverse: pant like a dog. You'll find you feel a bit nervy.

If you breathe each breath with full attention, you also narrow your mental focus. When you focus on just one thing, your mind lets go of a lot of other things—often dozens or hundreds of others. Consider that, as a routine, you think about one thought per second. That's about 3,600 per waking hour, or 60,000 thoughts per day. Cutting down on all the hustle and bustle can dampen a lot of tension and anxiety.

Why is this so? Because an overly busy mind runs away from the present moment. It flashes between the future and the past. At one moment, you're busy regretting a spat with a friend. The next, you're fretting over blowing the toast at your brother's wedding. Absorbed in the past and future, you lose track of the here and now. And that is where stress arises: from missing the joy of the present moment, getting lost in the past and future.

Paying attention to what you're doing right now is *mindfulness*. Just breathing—that's mindfulness! Just walking—that's mindfulness! Just eating—that's mindfulness! In mindfulness is relaxation. How many moments of the gazillion in your life have you lived mindfully? The more you can count, the better you probably feel.

Paying little attention to the present moment is *mindlessness*. Just regretting or fretting or wishing or expecting—that's mindlessness. In this chapter, you'll discover that stress comes from mindlessness. It comes from letting ourselves get swept away in an avalanche of thought and emotion. We may find many gems in that avalanche. Gems of wisdom, compassion, grace, creativity, and joy. We don't want to lose them. But we do want to dodge the hurtful stones of stressful thoughts that come whistling by at the same time.

Makings of a Stressful Life

In Maria Borne's life you might see hints of how stress disrupts the calm of your own life. Enlisting in the U.S. Army at nineteen, Maria became a one-star general's secretary in just four years. She won the job as a specialist when the general passed over a pool of other worthy candidates from the entire post. She handled all her boss's communications at division headquarters—and even ran the office on her own when he flew overseas. Maria had succeeded in a way many of her peers could envy.

But consider how, after "succeeding," she felt more stress. "Part of my job was to be the ideal soldier," she explains. So she trained to meet those high expectations. Among her top goals: to hold her top-ten spot in her group's physical-training test. To do so, she got up at 4:30 A.M., ran a loop through the neighborhood, spit-shined her boots, and donned a starched uniform. At 6:30 A.M., she did physical training. She worked out—doing lots of sit-ups and push-ups—for sixty to ninety minutes.

Now consider Maria's job duties. Under the army's open-door policy, all soldiers can call a general to air a gripe. They can call a general's secretary, too. Maria thus fielded five or six ticklish calls every day. Parents railed about daughters' or sons' treatment by officers. Soldiers pleaded for leniency after crimes or drunkenness. Maria listened. She absorbed the distress. Then she played back the reality of army regulations to her callers. "I was always the bearer of bad news," she says.

Maria didn't have a lot of control over her work. Does this sound familiar? A lack of control stresses all of us. In Maria's case, the stress was compounded by a huge workload. When soldiers needed answers, she had to rattle them off. If she couldn't, she had five minutes, tops, to produce them. "I had to be the fount of information," she says. She busied herself reading anything she could get her hands on about military regulation. She was frantic to keep up.

Maria worked, as many people do, in constant fear—the fear of not measuring up. And for Maria this was acute. "I was working in a fishbowl," she explains. "All eyes were on me." As the top secretary, she couldn't screw up. Everyone would see. Everyone would talk. Maria dreaded not meeting her goals. She feared defeat. She especially feared defeat in so visible a job.

We hope you don't have as stressful a job as Maria's. But you probably recognize some of your own patterns of stressful thinking. Like Maria, you may fasten your mind on meeting sky-high (too-high!) expectations. You may strive for control you can't secure. You may hunger for recognition. You may feel vulnerable. Or helpless. Or hopeless. Try as you may, you feel overwhelmed by second thoughts about the past and second-guessing the future.

In simpler terms, you may find yourself stuck with the same burden as Maria: "I was carrying all this stress and not putting it down," she says. "I could not relax."

How Your Mind Reels

You don't have to have a high-pressure job to feel stress and anxiety. Most people from all walks of life have to cope with stress. A Lou Harris poll found that nearly nine out of ten Americans experience "high" levels of stress. A report from Indiana University says that one quarter of Americans have felt they were on the verge of a nervous breakdown.

No wonder that among the twenty top-selling drugs in the United States are four for depression and anxiety.

But how can this be so? You may be familiar with surveys of people's well-being. These show consistently that most people are happy most of the time. And for the most part it doesn't matter if you're rich or poor, or from a rich or poor country (unless you're destitute). Most people report that they feel at least mildly happy. They say they are satisfied with work, marriage, health, finances, friendship.

But here's the catch: Counting yourself as happy doesn't mean you enjoy a life free of stress. No matter who you are, stress may get the better of you. As we've started to find with Maria, there's a simple reason: our minds often have a "mind" of their own. They get carried away. As novelist/essayist Virginia Woolf put it: "My own brain is to me the most unaccountable of machinery—always buzzing, humming, soaring roaring diving, and then buried in the mud."

When our minds get carried away in this fashion, they can sweep us into states of stress and anxiety—even when nothing in our lives appears upsetting. One reason is that our minds work so fast. They pile up thoughts at such a rapid clip that they can knock us silly in seconds. Scientist Mihaly Csikszentmihalyi notes that our mind can process seven items at once—items such as sounds, odors, images, or emotions like joy or anger. He notes further that we need only 1/18 of a second to process each item. The result is that we can process 126 pieces of information every second. That's 7,560 per minute, half a million per hour!

Our unconscious mind—out of sight but not, so to speak, out of mind—churns through information even faster.

Thousands of times faster. It is in the unconscious that we store habits of how to think, feel, and act. But we don't see the unconscious with more than dim awareness. We only see hints of it in puns, jokes, slang, dreams, and slips of the tongue. We also see hints as we repeat behaviors throughout our adult lives that we learned in early childhood.

Such capacity does the mind have! Neuroscientists estimate the human brain contains 100 billion neurons. Each neuron has 1,000 connections. Each connection fires on average 200 times per second, resulting in 20,000 trillion calculations per second! With such horsepower, the mind can easily produce all the action of a three-ring circus. Imagine the scene: In the left ring, we run old newsreels of childhood. We relive a game of tag, or we remember a scolding. In the middle ring, we concoct visions of the future. We win the most-valuable-employee award, or take in a movie. In the right, we track what we're doing right now. We're pedaling our bike through potholes in a rainstorm. All the while, we feel the brush of related feelings, thoughts, sensations, urges.

We may enjoy this circus. At least sometimes. It's titillating, after all. But the good circus acts always come with the bad. Sometimes they're overwhelmed by the bad. If you're under pressure at work, you may find this circus especially unpleasant. You may fret about all that could fail tomorrow or next week. You may worry about how your next project will affect your career. You may even lay awake nights in spite of recent successes.

You may find, in short, that your mind is wracked with negative thought. One businessman we know described this state colorfully: "I had this dog and cat fight in my head and I was in the middle of it," he said. "It felt like an infinite number of cats and dogs."

You may have exhausted yourself spawning thought that triggered just this kind of mental conflict. Instead of focusing on the here and now, you may have let your mind churn with useless cat-and-dog thinking. If so, you have to ask yourself: When you feel tired at the end of the day, are you tired from your job? Or are you tired from countless—needless—revolutions of your mind?

The "One-Minute Mind"

In trying to heal your mind, you will come upon a startling fact: When your mind runs out of control, it may *seem* like an infinite number of thoughts are running through it. But if you write them down, you'll find no more than several dozen. Our minds rarely spew forth as much original thought as we think. We're creatures of habit. Roughly nineteen out of twenty thoughts we think today are the same as those from yesterday.

Despite our huge potential for fresh thinking, our mind mostly repeats. Over and over. In spite of flashes of creativity, we largely step from one time-worn piece of mental turf to the next. We deepen decades-old ruts minute after minute after minute. At any given time, the best and worst of our thinking bubbles nonstop in our heads. The clairvoyant and confused, the generous and greedy, the loving and hateful, the courageous and fearful.

For all the variety, the perceptions that run through our minds each day are similar. The memories are similar. The urges, the emotions, the plans—they're all similar. If you pluck from your day one minute of thought, you may easily pluck a miniature of your whole life. This is the day-to-day mind. The everyday mind. The habitual mind. We call it the "one-minute mind."

The one-minute mind is a name for the mind that directs us along habitual pathways of thought. It bedevils us by putting us on negative tracks of thinking. It recycles painful memories. It guides us mindlessly into age-old behaviors. It is a mind that often runs at warp speed. We experience this mind all day, and we know it far less well than we think. And it is this mind—the one-minute mind—that fires the boilers of stress.

Take for a moment the mind of a teenager. You can imagine the types of thinking that play over and over: Can I make my grades? Do I like chemistry? Why am I even taking chemistry? Will I pass the class? Am I ever going to get a girlfriend (boyfriend)? Should I be in school? The one-minute mind runs back and forth over this and other territory time and time again. It can put any teen in a whirlwind of anxiety. Yet it often amounts to much ado about nothing.

Most of us, aware of the misery in the world, feel we have little to complain about. That's why so many of us report we're happy. But our minds are always attacking our contentedness. We feel hassled with doubt. We feel pestered over trifles. Even if we don't have a one-star general rapping on our desk, we let life's irritants, big and small, get under our skin. The result is that we have trouble becoming happy at our core. We feel stuck with a sense of dissatisfaction.

Falling into Habits of Mindlessness

Five More Breaths.   You are about to take the second step in learning to meditate. Settle again comfortably in your seat. Close your eyes. Draw in and expel five breaths. Once again, each time you breathe, feel your breath as if you've never felt anything like it before. Savor every instant. Enjoy the relaxation. Just breathe! And when you're done with your last mindful breath, read on.

What did you notice about your breathing this time? Was it once again relaxing? Probably so. Perhaps you noticed something else, too. Your mind bubbled with a few added thoughts. You may have compared your breathing this time with the last. You may have hoped you would enjoy each breath as much (or more!). Maybe you worried that you would enjoy it less. In short, your mind got in the way of your paying attention to your breathing.

In the language of meditation teachers, you couldn't breathe like a beginner. You didn't have "beginner's mind." Don't be dismayed. This is what you should expect. As a human, you've trained yourself too intensively to think like a perpetual motion machine to stop the engine of mental wandering. You simply can't help yourself. You think about all kinds of things almost all the time!

The one-minute mind acts out of habit. It shoots down railroad tracks traveled many times before. You don't give your mind permission to go there. You don't tell the mind which way to travel. Your mind chooses for you. As if against your will, it tickets you to a destination where you may or may not want to go.

Unfortunately, some tracks your conscious mind travels lead to places that threaten your health. They lead to the hostile territory of stress, anxiety, and other emotional pain. You find that one minute your mind runs on a productive track. So far, so good. But the next it jumps to a broken track that leads to destructive thinking. How do you know when you're on a good track or bad? There's no easy way to judge. But three tracks stand out as giving us some of the worst rides of our lives:

Judging

Our mind passes judgment on everything and everybody. We see our neighbor's smile, and we judge it safe. We hear the wind flutter the leaves, and we judge it with indifference. We see ice building up on our windshield, and we scowl with displeasure. No image, no sound, no thought, no odor passes through the gateway of our consciousness without the mind, as if with clipboard in hand, grading it as good, bad, or indifferent.

The mental track of judging gives us the ability to make good decisions. Good decisions make for a good life. But we all too easily slip into judging mindlessly. When we do, we often lapse into the unkind habit of denigrating ourselves and others. Remember Maria, the general's secretary. She judged herself against the standard of the perfect soldier. Her boss did the same. Her reward? Her mind got stuck on the track of negative self-talk. The track led to self-criticism. The criticism gathered momentum. It was hard to stop.

The track of judgment in turn leads to the track of blame. Once again, blame may be useful. If you're a judge or lawyer, placing blame helps do justice. But for the rest of us, it stirs up turmoil. Often needless turmoil that makes us burn inside.

The track of blame in turn leads to the track of anger. Once again, anger may not be unhealthy. But think about the possibilities. If you're angry with yourself, you cloud your thinking with guilt and self-doubt. If you're angry with others, you cloud it with righteousness and inflexibility. If you're angry enough, you may lash out—at your spouse, children, friends, colleagues. The possibilities for unhealthy action are endless.

Grasping

Grasping drives our lives. We spend nearly every waking minute going after what we want and avoiding what we don't want. Some people call this "the pleasure principle." Pursuing food, shelter, and sex assures our survival. Pursuing our dreams makes life worth living. But the pleasure principle has a downside. We can get on the track of following it mindlessly. We cede control to it. And in turn we lose control of our well-being.

The trouble with grasping is that we grasp without end. We always want more. And when we can't get it, we find we've run aground right where we started: with that persistent sense of dissatisfaction. We not only grasp at the makings of pleasure, we grasp at means to avoid displeasure. On the one hand we wish for ice-cream cones. On the other, we wish for smaller portions of broccoli.

What we learn on the grasping track is that we can't lead ourselves to lasting contentment. We enjoy temporary periods of it. But we can't string together enough of them to make a continuous stream. Just as life seems to burst with pleasure, the fun lurches to a halt. Our one-minute mind scans madly for the next bit of pleasure, but it often can't find anything within range. We then feel let down, and anxious about the future.

One thing we grasp for most is identity. We grasp urgently at ideas and things that make us who we are—whatever we feel we are. When we hold them close, we enjoy the feeling of strength. But enjoying our self-image is no different from enjoying other pleasures. We can't get enough, or get it long enough, to find permanent satisfaction. Letting ourselves mindlessly grasp at an identity puts us at risk of a very deep kind of stress. We ask, "Who am I?" And we feel empty when we don't have good answers.

"I didn't really know who I was. I didn't know quite where I was going." That's the kind of statement you would expect from someone looking back on his or her teenage years. Wanting to be one thing or another, teenagers all search for an identity. They look for the coursework, friends, and social life to define themselves. You probably remember doing this yourself. And you realize that you probably have never quite quit.

As we age, we may look even more avidly than before for an identity. We may search for jobs and homes and communities that reinforce our belief in what we are. This identity search, often frustrating, can whip up unceasing anxiety, whether we're sixteen or sixty. This is particularly so because we often end up mindlessly associating ourselves with things that give us no enduring peace.

Fearing

Among the most powerful of thought patterns is fear. We judge, then we fear. We grasp, then we fear. Along with looking for pleasure, the mind is constantly surveying for danger. In contrast to the pleasure principle, this might be called the danger principle. A thought arises, an image arises, and we ask, "What if?" We assess for risk, for danger. We can terrify ourselves this way.

A parallel track to fear is worry. Worry runs deep in all of our minds. In an informal poll, author and psychiatrist Robert Hallowell found that most people call themselves moderate to severe worriers. That doesn't mean people are not happy overall. But they're aware that so much is uncertain as life changes. So much can go wrong. We may not get something we want badly. We may lose it when we do get it. We may humiliate ourselves when that joke we told at a neighborhood party falls flat.

To be sure, we have to worry to some extent to survive. Fear and worry help us plan for crises and avoid disasters. But fear can overpower us. One of the worst fears is fear of aloneness. When this fear arises, it can prompt some disquieting questions: "Who cares about me? How am I connected? Why do I feel isolated?" Our minds can put us on this track at any moment, and this fear can become acute as we age.

Letting ourselves run mindlessly along the fearing track rattles us most often at times of change. Studies of managers, for example, show that they find five experiences most stressful: their first job, their first big promotion, moving to a new area, their first job as a boss, and retirement. Sound familiar? These are milestones we all worry about. The bogeyman of change shunts us onto the track of self-doubt: "What if they find out my weaknesses?" We feel a bit vulnerable, a bit helpless. We can't plan for all contingencies. We don't have full control.

If you're an employee, you may feel even more fearful than a manager. A boss, after all, controls your livelihood.

Recall Maria Borne. One day, a three-star general dropped in unannounced while her boss was in a briefing about a new computer system. Nobody was in the office. Should a general's office remain unmanned at any time? Of course not.

When Maria came back from lunch, she faced a commander spewing venom. Why is the office unmanned? What kind of soldier are you? How could you be so unprofessional? He didn't treat Maria to a kindly reprimand. He screamed at her. Says Maria: "I thought, oh my god, I'm getting kicked out of the army today! I'm ready to cry because I'm being yelled at, and I don't know why I deserve the blame."

Owing to the intense stress of this and other incidents, Maria began having severe headaches. They were so painful she cried. She had them almost every workday. "All I wanted to do was lay down with a cool rag on my head in a dark room," she says. Such is the power of fear in the work place. Of course, some of this fear comes from real events. But some arises from the mind's power to blow things out of proportion.

Judging, grasping, fearing. These are by no means the only mindless tracks that our one-minute minds push us onto. There are other "mental habits," like sadness, restlessness, boredom, fatigue, and grief. But as we look at our mindless patterns of judging, grasping, and fearing, we learn something new: Our one-minute mind is not always a wise, thoughtful, even-handed decisionmaker. It can be an impulsive, judgmental, and opinionated stooge. It acts fast. It acts by habit. It shoots from the hip. In other words, as each thought arises, it *reacts*. As if by reflex, it whisks us down age-old tracks to destinations unchosen, undesired, and stressful.

Does thinking have to be this way? Not at all. Another kind of mind is healthier. It is the mind that *responds*. It operates through mindfulness. It pays attention to what we're doing right now. It points us in wiser directions. It steers us clear of the land of stress.

Ruts and More Ruts

The fact is, we all have trouble doing anything mindfully. In the blink of an eye, we tend to take our mind off what we're doing. We start thinking about good things, bad things, irrelevant things. We lose track of what's going on. Judging, grasping, and fearing run amok, and we rush headlong to the brink of stress, and beyond. As we run in this unhealthy direction, we often derail at several common mental traps.

Catastrophizing

This is a way of saying we get caught in the trap of making mountains out of molehills. After a thought comes to mind, and after we react to it, the mind gets stuck on the reaction. We then succumb to tunnel vision. We block out other thoughts. We go on to build a small reaction into a giant one.

How does this work? Say you're in the post office one day. The clerk scowls at you. You don't know why. But you spend ten minutes picking yourself apart to find the flaw in your personality that caused the reaction. Now that's catastrophizing. (And you later find out the clerk just had car trouble on the way to work.)

Experiments by psychiatrist Aaron Beck showed that the mind reacts with tunnel vision naturally. Very hungry people tend to block stimuli not related to eating. Depressed people block out positive information about themselves. Panicky people block reasoning that would help them. Our minds distort reality. Fears, in particular, loom large. Fixating on fear, we view manageable problems as catastrophic.

That's not to say that some things shouldn't upset us. But we often worry ourselves sick by letting the small animals of stress turn into monsters. This was a lesson learned by Kevin Nuñez, a forty-year-old manager of an Oregon local utility company.

Kevin's story goes like this: He and his wife had become hooked on computer chat sessions. So often did they chat that they had three on-line names between them, one as a couple, two more as individuals. They became regulars in a chat room hosted in Philadelphia. They liked the people a lot, and chatted up a storm. On weekends they sometimes stayed on-line fourteen hours a day. They talked weather, they talked kids, they talked the time of day. They loved it.

But then Kevin felt his wife loved it a bit too much. He suspected she was making "inappropriate" chat with other men. Of course, the chat was on-line, with men she would never meet. But the chats roused Kevin's jealousy. Kevin became unnerved when his wife started clearing the screen when he walked into the room—and when other chatters hinted that his wife's chat had become a bit cozy.

Kevin talked it out with his wife. She promised to quit the chatting that bothered him. Still, she found it harmless. She couldn't resist going on-line. And then one day Kevin discovered on the computer browser's history list a new electronic greeting card from a chat-mate. It was just a generic animation of a rabbit saying "I love you." But Kevin blew up. In his tirade, he slammed an ashtray into the fire-place. He knocked knickknacks off the wall. Seething, he moved out that night and moved in with his mother. It would be another eight days before he decided to give the marriage another chance.

What Kevin admits today is that he got carried away. Sure, the chatting was offensive. But was it marriage-breaking? He recognized his wife's chat with other men played on his insecurities. By sitting often in meditation, he brought his anger back under control. He now says the most recent six months of his marriage have been the best in its entire ten years. Kevin recognized that his stress came not just from the offensive behavior. It came from his *reaction*. He fixated on it. He catastrophized.

Joyriding

Joyriding is the habit of spinning wild fantasies. It's daydreaming on overdrive. Throw a random thought into the engine of the mind, and the mind roars off on an adventure. Following the pleasure principle, it chases the interest of the moment—money, food, sex, sleep. Or following the danger principle, it seeks to avoid the fear of the moment, fear of hurt, of embarrassment, of loss, of grief.

Everybody can cite examples of their joyriding. Maybe you're in the basement one morning riding your stationary bicycle. You smell a hint of fuel oil in the air. The scent triggers a string of wild images: a pool of unignited fuel in the room. An explosion. Running out of the cellar. Streaking for the children's rooms with the flames shooting out the first-floor windows. Shaking the children awake. Tying bedsheets together. Urging the children out the windows into the hands of firefighters holding a tarp below. You can easily throw all these imaginings up on the screen of your mind in just a few seconds.

This is the mind on a joyride. Though sometimes helpful, and generally harmless, joyriding can become a trap. If you joyride mindlessly, your mind can railroad you quickly in the wrong direction. Then you're left grasping, wanting, getting tense. Or you're left fearing, feeling worried, getting stressed. Many of us fantasize all day long. Have you ever staged a soap opera around yourself? You imagine you have cancer, you rush to the hospital, your family grieves, you die and smell your flowers. This can seem silly. But the bout of stress that follows can be real.

One way we start joyriding is with "if-only" thinking. "If only I had a Corvette." "If only my boss weren't such a dictator." "If only my tennis serve were faster." We focus on what could be. And we can become tense over not having it, or start worrying we can't get it. Of course, we do want to improve ourselves. Joyriding can be a huge source of creativity. But we tend to dwell on the gaps. We see a chasm between us and where we want to be. We forget to enjoy the act of creating and building the bridge to our future. Stress mounts as we anticipate and plan. We lose the joy in the moment.

Going Overboard

When you let a few bad experiences shape your views of yourself, or when you let the exception prove the rule, you are going overboard. You make six lousy trades in the stock market. You lose 20 percent of your money. You conclude you can never make money (and maybe you can't). Your neighbor makes six winning trades in the stock market. She makes 20 percent on her money. You conclude that she can always make money (and maybe she can).

In any case, you suffer double the stress of this comparison by letting your mind bully you. You lose the money. That's problem enough. And then you fret over your abilities, your embarrassment, your self-esteem. That can be an even bigger problem. In other words, you get understandably stressed about the financial loss, but you get irrationally stressed about what you perceive as a fault in your personality.

Tyranny of Shoulds

This is the habit of expecting perfection from yourself and from others. Your mind dwells on the ideal. You judge yourself, as did Maria Borne, based on what you and others *should* do. You then react when the actual result differs. Often your reaction is unhealthy.

Craig Moser knows the tyranny of shoulds all too well. Craig was spectacularly successful in college. He ran track. He aced tests. He was the president of his fraternity. In short, he was a "hardcore overachiever, overproducer," he says. But he exhausted himself from working 14 to 18 hours a day. He had driven himself into the self-destructive habit of trying to achieve what he felt he *should* achieve. "The concept of fatigue didn't really enter in," he says. "I didn't want to feel it, didn't want to be aware of it."

Craig ran cross-country and track so much, ninety miles a week, that his body repeatedly broke down. As soon as it healed, he'd go at it again. He studied so much that he cut off some of his friends. He became tense enough that he lashed out at his girlfriend. He was driven not by the pleasure of achievement, but by the concept of the ideal.

We often project the tyranny of shoulds on others, especially as parents on our children. We then get frustrated when they don't rise to our standards. In a sense, we set other people up for failure. When those failures occur, we blame others and turn angry toward them. This sequence of thinking simply ignites stress. If, for example, we think our teenagers should leave the gas tank full, we fume when they don't. But are they the problem? Probably not. We may have simply enslaved ourselves with our personal tyranny of shoulds.

Besides catastrophizing, joyriding, going overboard, and the tyranny of shoulds, there are many other traps your mind may fall into. You may judge things in black and white, as all good or all bad. You may worry about every failure that affects your life, even though you may have had nothing to do with it. You may feel blue or negative one day, so you let your moodiness color everything negatively. Indeed, you may find that, if you step back, your mind acts like Wile E. Coyote: Forever hungry for realizing your dream of catching the roadrunners of life, your mind runs on just a few crazy tracks. And many of these tracks cause stress.

The habits of the one-minute mind take a toll on many of us. Sometimes a toll paid in days, months, or years of stress. As you learn to better cope with the reactive mind through meditation, you will learn to recognize your mental habits. And you will learn to put them aside, along with the one-minute mind.

How Stress Hurts

What is stress, anyway? Experts have trouble defining it. The fact is, stress, love, pain, and similar terms will always be vague. Suffice to say, stress is physical, mental, or emotional distress we have trouble adapting to. When we can't adapt, we get mentally and physically tense. The tension reveals itself in ways that simply don't feel good. The burning in your stomach. The knot in your shoulders. The ache in your forehead. The twitter in your intestines. But when push comes to shove, most of us figure we can always bear up under stress. We figure we won't die from it.

But experiments over the last hundred years show that we don't bear up as well as we think. The superficial feelings of strain often signal deeper harm to our bodies. It all starts with our physiology. At a certain threshold of stress, glands in our bodies release a cocktail of hormones. For early man, this cocktail was lifesaving. It aroused the body and mind to action. Woolly mammoth on the way? The cocktail gave man the energy to run for a cave.

The threats we face today aren't so grave. Still, our body reacts in the same way. The released hormones route more blood to our muscles. They focus our attention. They prepare us instantly to either fight or flee. In fact, scientists call the hormone release the "fight-or-flight response" (or an activation of the sympathetic nervous system). The more alarming the challenge to your survival, the more potent the hormone release. The release varies in strength with the object of our fear, our experience, our perception of control, and other factors.

Topping the list of ingredients in the cocktail are *epinephrine* and *norepinephrine*. (You may know them as *adrenaline* and *noradrenaline*, respectively.) With as little as a pinprick, nerve endings in the adrenal medulla, above our kidneys, release both of these hormones into the bloodstream. With a lag of a minute or two, the adrenal cortex, also above the kidneys, releases a hormone called *cortisol*.

As the two enter your bloodstream, your heart pounds. Your breath speeds up. Your blood pressure and metabolism jump.

Now what happens when just your catastrophizing one-minute mind causes stress? Even if the threat is only imaginary, your body triggers the fight-or-flight response. This may seem hard to believe. After all, the danger lies only in your head. But your body takes it for real. The alarm sounds. You get pumped full of hormones for action—even if you have nowhere to go, no action to engage your aroused body.

When these hormones are coursing through your body, you stay pumped up—and now feel physically stressed—even if you dismiss your crazy thoughts. Epinephrine and norepinephrine peak in your blood right away. They then last many minutes. (Their "half-life," or time to fall to half their initial concentration, is one to three minutes.) But cortisol peaks in your blood in fifteen to thirty minutes and lasts for hours. (Its half-life is seventy minutes.)

A good example of the fight-or-flight response commonly arises during public speaking. If you get nervous as you step before a crowd, you experience a tripling of epinephrine levels in fifteen minutes. These levels go back to baseline about fifteen minutes later. But if you can't shake stressful thoughts, your cortisol levels can stay high for a couple of hours. Only then do other hormones kick in and naturally cool an overheated system. The point is, each time you sound an alarm over a real or imagined fear, you flood your bloodstream with stimulants. And these stimulants last a lot longer than your momentary thoughts.

How can this affect you day to day? Take a page from the

life of Dot Smerciak, a sixty-one-year-old critical-care nursing supervisor. Not long ago, Dot found a typical set of
problems in the intensive-care unit. First, she discovered
that a nurse had made an error the night before. No fluid
was running through a patient's intravenous line. She fixed
the error and dealt with the nurse. Next she discovered that
she had to care for an alcoholic in withdrawal. He was
thrashing under leather restraints. His blood pressure was
soaring, and Dot knew his risk of stroke was rising.

Meanwhile, Dot handled administrative tasks. At one
point, she juggled three phone calls. All the while she had
to keep her other eye on some terribly ill patients. By 10
A.M., she says, "I had this tension through my scalp." Who
on earth wouldn't?

As was her habit, Dot extinguished this stress through
meditation. She does nearly every day. But she only found
her way to meditation after enduring more than her share
of fight-or-flight cocktails. Ten years ago, she routinely
went home with chest pains. Her shoulders and neck
tensed with stress. At night she would wake up suddenly. "I
wondered at first, is it my heart?" she recalls. "I hooked
myself up to the machine and could see that my heart was
fine. . . . I realized it was just plain stress and I had to relieve
it."

In Dot's line of work, stressful events come with the territory. Still, she shows that our minds, not our circumstances, work us into a state of alarm. And we can use our
minds to work ourselves out of that awful state. She shows,
too, how persistent is our one-minute mind. Day in and day
out, it takes us down the same tracks of stressful thinking.
By letting our minds run mindlessly, we are challenged
daily to keep our inner alarm silent.

Stress Sickness

Testing Your Alarm.   You are about to take the third step in learning to meditate. Settle comfortably as before. Close your eyes. Let muscle tension drain from your face, your shoulders, your arms, your legs. Now visualize in detail an event that made you fearful. Troubles with your boss. Speaking in public. Difficulties with sex. Arguing with a friend. Now scan your body. Where do you feel the fear physically? In the gut? Forehead? Shoulders? Feel how it moves, reshapes, grows, shrinks.

If you pay close attention in this one-minute meditation, you will experience the link between mind and body firsthand. If, say, you relived a stressful speech, you may have felt your shoulders hunch, your voice box contract. If you relived sharp words you had with vandals who smashed your mailbox, you may have felt heat in your chest, clenching in your jaws. If so, you will have felt the connection between stress created in your mind and illness-in-the-making in your body.

If you have any doubt about the harmful effect of stress on your health, here are a few statistics that will clarify the story. In a study of 46,000 employees tracked for three years, those reporting stress racked up 46-percent higher health-care costs. In another study, researchers estimated that three out of four health-care visits are for stress-related symptoms and illnesses.

Your Heart

Decades of research show that stress harms our heart and blood vessels by raising blood pressure. By repeatedly boosting your blood pressure temporarily, you risk keeping it up permanently. Doctors used to tell people they had "high blood pressure" when their systolic number (high end) rose and stayed above 139 and their diastolic (low end) rose and stayed above 89. But today we know that letting your pressure rise from even lower levels can sharply boost your risk of dying from heart disease. One large recent study suggests that you put yourself in significantly greater danger as your systolic pressure goes up by just ten points or your diastolic goes up by just five.

High blood pressure damages the arteries and leads to hardening (clogging) of the arteries with fat. Clogged arteries in the heart cause heart cells to die, causing a heart attack. Clogged arteries in the brain cause brain cells to die, sometimes impairing thinking and moving. This can happen suddenly, in a stroke, or slowly, in vascular dementia. The danger of driving up blood pressure is greatest for people with heart disease.

For many people, high blood pressure comes straight from the stressful lives they lead. Louisa Keniston, forty-three, dates her high blood pressure to starting her business. Emigrating from the Bahamas, she had normal blood pressure. Eight years later, she opened a bakery. She makes rolls, pita, and beef, turkey, vegetable, tofu, and spinach patties. She sells retail, and also to restaurants. Louisa's bakery is a success.

But Louisa has struggled with the hardships of all start-up businesses. Her equipment doesn't always work. Help is hard to find and costly to keep. Financing is scarce yet critical to business solvency. To keep on top of things, she works from 9 A.M. to 8 P.M. "It took so much out of me building the business," she says. Part of what the business was taking out of her was her health. Her blood pressure skyrocketed to 160/110.

"I was under stress left, right, and center," Louisa says. But she caught her problem in time. When medication failed to work, she began to meditate twice daily. She cut her blood pressure to 130/72. But others are not so lucky. High blood pressure kills more than 40,000 people a year in the United States. No doubt many of those who died failed to find a way to cope with stress before it was their undoing.

Your Breathing

In many people, stress takes its worst toll on another vital part of the body: the respiratory system. By now you have a first-hand feel for the link between mind and breathing. Breathing seems to offer a bridge between mind and body. Research confirms the bridge really exists. In lab experiments, when people voluntarily slowed their breathing and took bigger breaths, their anxiety declined. When they hyperventilated (breathed quickly and deeply) voluntarily, they stirred up symptoms of anxiety. Not surprisingly, people under stress may hyperventilate without even knowing it.

Researchers linked breathing and stress long ago. In 1886, Sir James Mackenzie brought a paper rose under glass to a young asthma patient who experienced asthma attacks from real roses. The fake rose also triggered an attack. This was the first of many simulated-stress experiments. Over the years, these showed that lab-induced stress tightens breathing in one out of five asthmatics. So sensitive are some people that they suffer an attack from just *imagining* a strong emotion.

Does stress cause the onset of asthma as an illness? A lot of research says it does. In one study of more than 400 asthmatics, two out of five named stress as a major factor triggering the onset of their asthma. Just about the same number said stress played a secondary role. So we know that stress can be harmful for those people susceptible to asthma.

But what if you're not susceptible to asthma? It turns out that if you let yourself get stressed out, you become a target for coughs and colds. In several remarkable studies, researchers asked people to sniff nasal drops loaded with different cold viruses. In one study, nearly 400 people participated. The rate of infections rose steadily with the subjects' stress levels. In other words, cold bugs attack stressed-out people much more than others.

Immunity

What with stress undercutting the fight against the common cold, you might guess the reason: Stress weakens our germ-fighting systems. You might guess, too, that with hobbled germ defenses, we might fall prey to all kinds of sickness. In truth, scientists suggest this is true, but they can't prove it. They do know that stress makes us "immunodepressed." They just don't know if this weakening of defenses is enough to make us ill.

Still, consider some details from research. In one study of stressed-out students before exams, the number of natural killer cells and T lymphocytes fell significantly. Natural killer and T-cells are key to fighting tumors. "Mitogen response"—a related and more important immune-system measure—also fell. In another study, similar results turned up after medical students took national board exams: Their immune system took six weeks to get back to normal. What is clear is that stress harms the battle-readiness of the immune system.

Mental Illness

When stressed, we sweat and flush. Our backs ache. Our hearts race. We have trouble sleeping. We may become irritable, anxious, panicky, fearful, angry, depressed. But again, research fails to show that stress causes mental illness. Of course, some people seem to thrive as they respond to stress. But for most of us, enduring too much stress can make us feel like an illness has gotten hold of us.

This was the case with Maria Borne, the army specialist. Trying to whip her stress, she exercised more at the gym. She tried midday napping. She went to church. She tried sitting and "vegetating." "I was definitely on a search," she says. "I was trying anything I could to relax." Feeling like she couldn't solve the problem on her own, she says finally, "I thought I was actually depressed."

Maria went to the army's mental health unit. She felt she just couldn't boost her sense of well-being. The doctors thought she was right. They even wanted to admit her to the hospital for depression. But Maria resisted. She felt the diagnosis didn't quite fit. It was at this time she began to meditate, at first just two minutes or so at a time. At work, she would watch for a lull and then snatch two or three minutes to sit in her car. "I'd listen to myself breathe in and out," she says. "It brought peace of mind for me. . . . It was like coming out of a haunted house. . . to realize it's all in my mind." Meditation helped ease her stress and, in turn, raised her spirits.

Other Physical Problems

Research links stress to many other conditions—from headaches to epilepsy. But the data to date fail to show that stress alone *causes* these ailments. What we do know is that doctors routinely document that stress and these disorders coincide. Headaches often begin with stress, and get worse as stress rises. Certainly Maria Borne and many other people experience headaches related to stress.

Irritable bowel syndrome is a common problem that accounts for 2.5 million doctor visits a year. It causes pain in the abdomen and changes in bowel-movement frequency and form. Why this happens we don't know for sure. But some scientists maintain there is a link to stress. In one experiment, researchers stressed people by immersing their hands in cold water or giving them a stressful interview. Movement in the colon changed markedly.

Researchers will be working for years to uncover the secrets of how stress contributes to illness. For now we can say that the picture painted by current research shows the mind and body interact very closely. Stress may begin with circumstances beyond your control—with a difficult boss, a high-pressure job, the rigors of growing up, with changes in family life. But it may also come from within, from imaginings of your own mind.

Either way, your one-minute mind can send you spinning into a spiral of unhealthy thinking. By understanding the mind, by seeing how it can react mindlessly, we take the first step in eliminating stress.

Pen and Paper

Clocking Your Stress. Draw the face of a clock on a piece of paper. Now divide the clock up, like a pie, into pieces. Each piece should represent the proportion of time you estimate that you spend during a normal day in different kinds of thought. Label the pieces with the subject of your thinking, such as "job," "food," "partner," "sex," "kids," "money," and so on. The face of your clock shows how many seconds of the average minute (or how many minutes of the average hour) you spend engaged in different areas of thinking.

Now crosshatch, or shade, each piece in which your thinking was in the past or the future. These are the times when your mind was not in the "present moment." You were on a track of mindlessness instead of mindfulness. This is the face of your one-minute mind. If you're like most of us, your face is mostly dark. Adding light to that face is the task ahead of you.

2

The One-Minute Escape

The soul grows by subtraction, not addition.

—HENRY DAVID THOREAU

> Turning Outward. Close your eyes once again. For one minute, think about all the things you desire. How about a cold drink? A hug from a friend? Five minutes to enjoy a cigarette? Half an hour to watch TV? A fresh apple fritter? An afternoon to doze on the beach? An evening to sleep with someone you love? An hour to play tennis? A lifetime in a new and more exciting place? Let your mind run for sixty seconds. If you like, write each item down.

If you're like most people, you can probably think of a dozen or more things you desire. And nearly every item on your wish list has one thing in common: It expresses a yearning for something outside yourself. We call this the one-minute escape. Desiring this escape is a universal compulsion. It is the longing to find contentment by turning outward. Rarely do we think first to turn inward.

31

One-minute escapes are our antidotes for the discomfort of the one-minute mind. In search of pleasant sensations, we snack on chips. Or pour a drink. Or take a drug. Or put on some music. Or engage in sex or masturbate.

Or we throw ourselves into work or play. We try to make a name for ourselves in our jobs. Or we practice fly tying or roller blading or needlepoint. Or we volunteer at the hospital or soup kitchen or grade school. By engaging our mental faculties, we bring order to our one-minute mind. We redirect our runaway mental engine onto a healthy and productive track. And we feel fulfilled.

A one-minute escape is our first impulse in dealing with stress. It is the mother's milk of the moment. And it often does us good. The question is how much good? For how long? *To the exclusion of what else?*

To subdue stress, we engage in one-minute escapes all the time. We find they numb the stress for at least a little while. But they are interim antidotes, like the pills we pop. And they come with a downside. They point us the wrong way for enduring stress relief. They may point us away from mindfulness of the present moment.

One Man's Escape Route

Josh Bellemore learned how we can trap ourselves by pursuing the one-minute escape. At twenty-seven, Josh had the blues. He felt sad, stressed, and anxious. But after many years of feeling this way, he was sure he had found the way to completely subdue these awful feelings—a radically new diet. A friend had explained how hypoglycemia, a low blood-sugar condition, causes depression. That explanation seemed to fit his periodic waves of down-and-out feelings.

Josh was sold on the diagnosis—and the treatment. He ate whole-grain millet in the morning. He ate seeds, nuts, and fruits at lunch. He ate a big garden salad loaded with vegetables at dinner. He never ate sugar because he was convinced that sugar was his problem. "I lived on this diet religiously," he says, and in a year and a half he dropped from a weight of 160 pounds to 130.

And he was pleased. The diet seemed to pump more joy into his life. Meanwhile, events started to turn in his favor. A painter of houses and aspiring professional guitarist, Josh played the guitar for as many as sixteen hours a day for several years. Then a contact in the music industry told him that he was as good as the best recording artists. Josh cut a tape with another musician. He wrote his own songs. He began to feel he was moving in on his just reward. "I was going to be a famous rock star," he says.

But alas, after eighteen months, he suddenly felt worse than ever. The down-and-out feelings came back. He had to admit that the diet was a sham. "It didn't work at all," he says.

Although the details of Josh's life are unique, his search for the contented life is a lot like all of ours. To deal with stress and anxiety, we energetically seek creature comforts. Or give in to enticing distractions. Or take creative cures. "I did every conceivable health food and nutritional thing you could do," Josh says. "I was desperate to figure it out."

But as one wise meditation teacher told Josh, "You are like a moth at night. You fly over and over into a hot light bulb. Your way of thinking repeatedly burns you." He would only stop burning himself when he saw his pattern of escape. And it was with the help of meditation that he did see this pattern.

Good Escapes (But Not Good Enough)

We're all a bit like moths. We spend a lot of time going after things outside ourselves. Whatever it is that attracts our minds and bodies, we grasp after them. In some ways, we find contentment. In fact, we find enough satisfaction that we redouble our efforts to hunt down the outside solution of the moment. As it turns out, many of these solutions are healthful, even if not enduring.

A set of experiments led by psychologist Mihaly Czikszentmihalyi shows just which escapes give people the most pleasure. The people participating in the experiments wore electronic pagers throughout the day. At random intervals, the pagers would go off. The people would then write down what they were doing and how they felt. The results showed that they felt most happy and relaxed at mealtimes. The simple lesson? Eating is a great stress reliever.

No wonder we like to snack and dine. It fills the stomach and lifts the spirit. Of course, redoubling your efforts to find joy in food may redouble your size. You may then run a health risk from weight and obesity problems. But you can see that if eating is so relaxing, you should spend more time at the table. You don't have to eat more, just eat more mindfully. And remember: While fast food isn't great for your health, fast eating may be worse.

Why is eating so calming? In part because tasting, chewing, and filling our bellies satisfy our hunger. In part because these actions make us feel comforted. Touching our lips to things that have pleased us since birth is especially enjoyable. We also enjoy sitting down with company. Coffee breaks give us pleasure not just from sugar, caffeine, and warm liquids. They help us reconnect with people and ourselves.

It's no surprise, then, that another healthy relief from stress is talking with others. Who wants to be left out, or left alone? We all fear it. Chatting keeps our fears at bay. As we give voice to our anxious feelings, we can escape stressful thinking. Consider the research with pagers. The results show that teenagers find socializing as the number one activity for arousing positive feelings. (For teens, eating was number two.)

Another healthy stress reliever is sex. Our genetic programming assures that as we engage in foreplay and intercourse, we focus more naturally on the present moment. We become more absorbed than in most other acts in daily life. Fears of the past, and worries about the future, recede into the background. Our bodies naturally build with sexual energy. During orgasm, we tap the energy and release tension naturally.

Of course, as with eating and socializing, sex can become habitual, compulsive, or destructive. If so, it may reflect stress as much as quell it. Sex may even become a means to avoid true intimacy. It may be impersonal, or even abusive or violent. If so, it becomes an escape of an unhealthy kind. In a healthy, loving relationship, a couple unites mind and body. They engage in sex to fulfill each other, and create a sense of complete intimacy.

The Way of Exercise

No matter what else you do in life, if you're stressed, you should get exercise. If you play a competitive sport, all the better. By engaging in sports, you cultivate mindfulness without even trying. What's more, during any exercise your body releases a number of chemicals which enhance well-being. One class of these is *endorphins*, natural opiates, which reduce pain and calm the body. Another is *serotonin*, which enhances contentment. For some people, exercise may be a cornerstone of stress-relieving therapy.

Richard Benz, fifty-nine, had worked for twenty years in a northeastern university's physical plant. He had been happy in his job. He supervised the maintenance of air conditioning, gas boilers, and the power system. And he had gotten good performance reviews. But a new boss turned his working world upside down. This new boss was young, thirty-something, eager to hire people his own age. He wanted computer-savvy people, too, and early on revealed contempt for Richard and his meager technological skills.

"When he came on board," says Richard, "he wanted to replace certain people on the job, and I was one of them." Thus began a seven-year standoff between the two men. In the first year, the boss transferred Richard to a lousy job. He also gave Richard lousy performance reviews. In response, Richard took a lot of time to learn spreadsheets, however hard the challenge of learning to use a new tool.

"He was very critical of me," says Richard. "Regardless of what I did, it never satisfied him. . . . He tried to find ways to constantly keep pressure on me so that I might quit."

Under the strain, Richard started to get headaches. His gut hurt so much he felt he was getting ulcers. His neck muscles tensed like violin strings. He sometimes stopped his truck on the way home from work to pull himself together. At home, he says, "I would tell my wife I just needed to be left alone for a while; I wasn't ready to talk or communicate." He would sit back in his recliner, relax, and pray.

"My mental attitude toward my boss was such that I did not like the thoughts going through my mind," he says. "I got to the point that I hated to go to work." His only relief was exercise. He played racquetball so aggressively, almost angrily, that he burned through his pent-up frustration. He'd then take a long, hot shower. For ten to fifteen minutes, he'd let the water pound on his aching neck.

Perhaps you've worked under some of the same strains as Richard. And maybe you've come to the same conclusion. As much as exercise helps, it cannot stop all the stress. Even after five years of trying to cope with the stress, each time Richard heard his boss's voice, he says, "I could almost feel my scalp crawl." A devout Christian, he even took to praying for his boss. For two years, he prayed that his boss would get a good job elsewhere.

Richard finally eased the grip of stress on his life by learning meditation. He now meditates each evening and takes periodic three- to five-minute breaks during the day. Along with people like Josh, Richard found that stress-relieving strategies from outside ourselves offer good therapies. Exercise, eating, sex, and chat cool the heat of a mind on fire. But they all fall short in putting it out for one key reason: They offer only one kind of cure, a cure from the outside.

As a variation of the old joke goes, we often look for our lost keys under the lamppost. Why? Because that's where the light is. We may forget entirely to look in the unlit byways. We can't see there. But in the case of stress, the keys aren't where the light is. They are often where we have shed little light before. They're in the shadows of the mind, in our habits.

Driven to Distraction

The One-Minute Challenge.   Close your eyes again. For the next minute, or about the time it takes for a dozen breaths, train your attention entirely on your breathing. Become absorbed in the rise and fall of your abdomen. Think of nothing else! See if you can stay absorbed. If your mind drifts, make a mental note of what you see or think.

How did you do? Unless you're a saint or guru, your chances of keeping your mind solely on your breath are slim to none. That's perfectly normal. Remember from Chapter 1: Your mind works hard to stay busy. You've trained your whole life to make it work that way. You can't stop it for a minute, or even for half a minute after much practice. You cannot stop your thoughts. You probably never will.

But what did you note mentally? Perhaps a thought about succeeding or failing? Or about your resolve to meet the challenge? Or about feeding your growling belly with french fries? Or about Richard taking a racket to his boss's hide? If you did note your thoughts, you really succeeded: You began to learn about your mind. How it springs into action. So quickly. So sneakily.

If you examine your mind, you'll find that you've fallen into the habit of letting distractions capture much of your attention. Even when you try to concentrate, your mind launches in a dozen directions. It distracts you when you're having fun; it distracts you when you're not. It distracts you when you're stressed; it distracts you when you're calm. In bed, on the phone, in the pool, on the ball field, in a con-cert, on a deadline. The mind is always hollering to get you to move on to something new.

Even when you purposefully pause to soak in the moment—at long last enjoying a minute of free time on the weekend—your mind still distracts you with other thoughts. In fact, you may notice your habit of distraction most at such times. In the emptiness of a free moment, the mind often uses a magnifying glass on itself. It pops the big questions about who we are and how we belong. Of course, if we don't have the answers, our minds can rush down an unhealthy track—plunging us into depression or anxiety.

That's why so many of us learn to distract ourselves. We play mental games. We get a drink. We pick our nails. We light a cigarette. We surf the Net. We face the emptiness of the moment as little as we can. Many people have a hard time with solitude. They face their naked selves then. They don't have work schedules to order their lives.

Of course, there's nothing wrong with many distractions. In fact, they may help you feel less stressed. At the right time, they're a great escape. Studies show that distractions help us all to cope with stress. One of the simplest exam-ples: In an experiment, nineteen- to forty-eight-year-old dental patients were given music to play through earphones while their cavities were being filled. They reported signif-icantly less pain, less discomfort, and a sense of more con-trol than a group that didn't hear music.

But the trouble with distractions comes when they become habitual one-minute escapes—when we flee from the present moment as if by reflex. At the extreme, we become slaves to compulsions or addictions. Compulsive gamblers, for instance, go to the track and fantasize about winning back all their lost money (and more). Their one-minute minds take over, and their thoughts blot out all their mental discomfort.

The Culture of Busyness

One risk we run by indulging in distractions is that we learn to cope with stress with busyness. The media, of course, often praise busyness. Glamorous people "multitask." They listen to the radio, check stocks, drink coffee, download songs, chat on the phone—all at the same time, and while driving. If we're adept enough, the media seem to tell us, we can put together a continuous stream of happiness. No gaps need remain in our access to pleasure. Such busyness can feel great—for a while. But running our lives on fast forward can also help us hide stress from ourselves.

Some people will argue that busyness is good. That busy minds drive creativity. That creativity drives fulfillment. That fulfillment is necessary to live a satisfied life. Maybe true. But if we cultivate busyness as a way to avoid learning more durable ways of acquiring well-being, we may have to rethink our approach to life.

"Don't just sit there, do something!" someone says. And we jump to action. But why do we often prize action over inaction? Why do we feel the impulse to act? Is it industriousness? Or is it a compulsion to distract ourselves? When you feel too busy, you might ask yourself, "Does my stress come from busyness? Or does my busyness come from an attempt to camouflage stress?" The last thing you want is to feel enslaved by the feeling that doing something, anything, is better than doing nothing.

"After a man arrives in heaven," an old joke begins, "he gets a chance to talk with God. 'God,' he says, 'I prayed and prayed all my life. Why didn't you ever answer?' And God says, 'I tried to reach you, but the line was always busy.'" If your line is always busy, it may be time to think about hanging up once in a while.

Acquiring Versus Letting Go

Most of us find TV relaxing. Research shows that people watching TV reach high levels of relaxation with very little effort. TV ranks near the top in relaxing people compared to everything else they do during the day. That's a pretty big endorsement for TV watching. It should cheer the average American, who lives in a household that keeps the TV on for seven hours a day.

But TV can become an unhealthy escape. If you watch the tube compulsively to distract yourself, you may be simply hiding your stress. In place of one-minute mental ramblings, you install stories produced in Burbank and Hollywood. In some cases, you may fall into the category of a "television addict," as do about one of every ten people. Self-described addicts use TV to distract themselves from unpleasant thoughts, regulate their moods, and fill time. Students calling themselves TV addicts are more unhappy, anxious, and withdrawn than other viewers.

TV ads reinforce the habit of looking outside ourselves for contentment. They imply that you can deal with every problem with a product or service. If you fall under the spell of this Madison Avenue logic, you let consumption become more than a way to serve your worldly needs. You let a "shop 'til you drop" habit become a way to repress anxiety. In extreme cases, you can come to depend on consumption. As many as five of every one hundred people are compulsive buyers. They shop to give themselves an emotional lift, repair hurt feelings, improve their sense of self-worth.

They're usually people with low self-esteem, depression, anxiety, or frustration.

Of course, everyone knows you cannot shop your way to happiness. But the deeper lesson is this: You cannot solve the ills of the one-minute mind by *acquiring* something, or *doing* something. You have to look at an alternative, namely solving problems by *letting go*. By *not doing*.

Distractions are a godsend at times. What would we do without a few diversions to break the rigor of life? When distractions subdue stress, they are harmless. But when they turn us away from the path of stress relief, they fog our sense of how to find the joy of the here and now.

From Good Escape to Bad

Feeling the Need. Close your eyes. Let the muscle tension drain from your face, your shoulders, your arms, your legs. Now visualize in detail something you crave. A cola. A cigarette. A kiss. A breath of sea air. The stronger the craving the better. Now scan your body from the head down. Where do you feel the craving physically? Mouth? Belly? Groin? Feel how the sensation moves, reshapes, and changes in size or texture.

If you've tuned into the most subtle sensations in your muscles and gut, you'll feel again the physical connection between mind and body. In the same way you felt the muscle tension of fear in the last chapter, you'll feel a physical urge to satisfy craving. You may feel your muscles gently contract in your jaw. Or a vague craving feeling in your organs.

These shadowy sensations follow from thoughts in the one-minute mind. Just as fearful thoughts lead to the physical fight-or-flight reaction, craving thoughts lead to physical urges in your muscles and gut. You can see—and feel— how the one-minute mind moves you physically toward one-minute escapes.

Along with escapes that are generally healthy, these urges can lead to escapes that generally are not. Escapes like using tobacco, alcohol, and drugs. Using many substances in moderation won't harm you. And they may quell stress temporarily. But, again, they don't help you deal with stress for the long haul. They are one-minute sedatives for the one-minute mind.

Recall the story of college student Craig Moser. Craig was the star student, cross-country runner, fraternity president. On the outside, he seemed to ride high and easy on life. He looked like a success story in the making. And in fact Craig has gone on to become a lawyer. He is now clerk to a federal judge. At twenty-nine years old, he has won the trust of a judge to juggle 800 cases at a time.

But in college, Craig would let small setbacks get the better of him. The workings of his one-minute mind—the "tyranny of shoulds"—would lead him to drink. Craig didn't recognize his problem at first. But as time went on, he saw a clear pattern: First he would get a poor grade on a test or essay. Next he would interpret the grade as a lack of praise for his value as a person. Third, he would feel inferior. Fourth, he would decide he had to "blow off steam." And finally, he would search for an escape, and the escape would always be the same.

Says Craig, "I would go out and get liquored up with my buddies." He reassured himself with the thought: "I'll feel better afterwards."

Craig was caught in a one-minute escape. His pattern of thinking is common to many tobacco, drug, and alcohol abusers. Craig's beliefs about himself and drinking spurred a craving. Craving spawned an urge. The urge spurred action. And Craig would take action that followed an unfortunate but time-honored college tradition: drowning the one-minute mind in alcohol.

Through it all, Craig didn't understand the root cause: faulty thinking. "It was just a thing I did," he says, "and how people knew me."

In hindsight, Craig saw that the bad feeling of inferiority and angst came from fear. Fear of bad grades. Fear of rejection. Fear of not reaffirming his identity. He used alcohol to chase away those bad feelings. Only after time did he change. Craig eased his stress with meditation. The meditation helped him see that a sequence of mental shenanigans led him to drink. But at the start, all he knew was that he just couldn't stop himself from drinking.

People who drink, smoke, and take drugs often tell stories like Craig's. They escape into substance abuse because they feel vulnerable in some way. They judge themselves helpless, inept, or as failures. They feel alone or disconnected. They think of themselves as unloved, different, rejected, or socially defective. These kinds of core feelings often lead to the risky alternatives of alcohol, drug, and nicotine use. And these feelings come from thoughts that begin in the one-minute mind.

From Escape to Addiction

In schools, in work places, in every part of society, people use and abuse drugs, alcohol, and tobacco. One of every eight adults in the United States is an alcoholic. One in four is addicted to nicotine. One in seventeen abuses illicit drugs such as marijuana. The problem touches every corner of society. It comes home in almost every family. Though we don't know all the exact roots of the problem, stress certainly contributes to it.

In a study of more than 7,000 households, men in high-stress jobs (high mental demand and low control) were twenty-seven times more likely to abuse alcohol than men in low-stress jobs. In a survey of 12,000 workers, nearly half of those in high-stress jobs were smokers, compared to a third in low-stress jobs. When you work or live under stress, you're at risk of giving into unhealthy one-minute escapes.

Recall Maria Borne. In trying to fight the stress of working in a work-place pressure cooker, Maria tried all kinds of things—extra exercise, napping, church, even "vegetating." When nothing seemed to work, she turned to something else: She indulged in three-day drinking binges on Thursday, Friday, and Saturday nights. She drank tequila and beer, weekend after weekend. "I'd party until I was ready to go to sleep," she says.

The link between stress and drugs may not be so direct for other people. Many people start using drugs simply for pleasure. Physician Andrew Weil even argues that we are born with an urge to use drugs (and smoke and drink) to achieve "altered states of consciousness." The drive is like hunger or sexual desire. It is another attempt to find peace of mind.

But a harmless urge to sample drugs for pleasure can degenerate into a harmful pattern of abuse. The well-known psychiatrist Aaron Beck outlined the reasons why recreational drug users can gradually become drug abusers. They use them to relieve anxiety, stress, and tension. To boost morale. To find a means to connect regularly with a group. In other words, they use them to escape from the challenges of the one-minute mind.

Abuse can lead to addiction. By definition, you're addicted when you use a substance heavily, while developing both tolerance and withdrawal symptoms. When you reach this state, as Beck has shown, your mind runs along a track of thinking that's hard to leave. It's a track that runs in a vicious circle—the more times you go around, the more distressed you become.

In simple terms, the spiral goes like this: Stress and anxiety prompt substance abuse (of alcohol, cocaine, marijuana, and other substances). Abuse creates personal problems (job loss, family strife, debt, and so on). Personal problems fuel more stress and anxiety. The stress and anxiety lead to more abuse.

Beck, a pioneer in therapy for addiction, notes seven abnormal beliefs that develop among people dependent on drugs, alcohol, tobacco, and even overeating. The beliefs could be phrased as follows:

"I need the substance to stay balanced."
"It will improve my thinking and social functioning."
"It will be fun and exciting."
"It will energize me and give me more power."
"It will soothe me."
"It will relieve my boredom, anxiety, tension, and depression."
"Unless something is done to satisfy the craving and neutralize distress, it will go on or worsen."

These kinds of beliefs can run wild in the one-minute mind. They arise not at random, but become habits, as the mind rushes time and time again down the same unhealthy track. They become the mental kindling that feeds the fires of cravings and urges, and leads to one-minute escapes that harm us.

An Escape of (Poor) Choice

An example of someone caught in the worst kind of spiral is Cathy Ardin, a single, twenty-eight-year-old college student. After graduating from high school, the rebellious third sister in a family of seven, she made her way from Houston to Miami. There she fell in love with Chris. Over their ten years together, Cathy and Chris traveled often. They loved the life of the road. They hitchhiked. They backpacked. Cathy set aside any thought of goals, college, or career.

But over the years she became intensely anxious. Her life had become riddled with drug use. Chris was addicted to methamphetamine. "Meth" is an illegal drug, a stimulant, also known as crank. It has swept urban and rural America as a top drug of addiction. (Ecstasy, another amphetamine, has rapidly taken hold.) Chris sold meth to support his and Cathy's lifestyle. Cathy began to deal with stress with some of the one-minute escapes we've described. She bought whatever she wanted—clothes, makeup, more drugs. She ate whatever and whenever she wanted. The distraction and eating eased her anxiety, but she gained fifty pounds.

When Cathy did return to school, she used meth to help her study. The drug made her feel strong and whole, and "helped" her and Chris focus to be able to get much more done. Cathy, however, became dependent on meth. She'd take the drug and get high. So far, so good. But when she came down, after twelve to twenty-four hours, she experienced mood changes and an unpleasant craving. So she took more meth as the solution to feeling bad. Over a couple of years, Cathy spiraled downward. Her life deteriorated to an almost constant state of severe anxiety and depression.

Drug-dependent users like Cathy often reach a crisis. Only then can they crawl back from the abyss. In Cathy's case, when Chris couldn't get meth, he began to punch her. When this kept up, she informed him she was leaving him. He beat her so severely the state intervened to pay for therapy for physical and emotional abuse. This intervention was Cathy's salvation. The therapy broke the cycle of addiction. And Cathy began using meditation to calm herself and control her one-minute mind.

Cathy is an extreme example. But her pattern of addiction is not. Users are so convinced of the benefits of drug use that they find it hard to break the habit. Whether they use meth, cocaine, alcohol, heroin, marijuana, or another drug, they hold strong beliefs about the "good times" ahead. Typically, they believe drugs will give them pleasure, improve their sexual performance, make them feel more powerful and assertive, or ease stress and tension. These beliefs become ingrained. So ingrained that they spur urges that, to the addict, seem to arise on their own.

Addiction can lead to illness, of course. Smoking causes lung, bladder, and other cancers, emphysema, and heart disease. Cocaine is linked to cardiac arrest, stroke, respiratory collapse, high blood pressure, and infection. Methamphetamine leads to severe depression. Alcohol, arguably the worst of all drugs, damages the liver, pancreas, gastrointestinal tract, and cardiovascular, immune, endocrine, and nervous systems. What's amazing is that many of these illnesses, which lead to premature death, can start simply with the errant workings of the one-minute mind.

The Way Out

In the big picture, all one-minute escapes are much the same. They appeal to us because we're hooked on the habit of looking outside for relief. This is just as true in the case of Josh Bellemore, the nuts-and-grains dieter, as it is for Cathy Ardin. When we, as humans, seek relief, we often forget the most obvious place to search: in the mind of the person we see in the mirror.

So in a sense we can all become addicted to the one-minute escape. But we can also make the decision to turn away from it—and turn toward mindfulness. When Cathy did, she started on a road to recovery. When Craig and Maria did, they turned their backs on the risks of alcohol abuse and took control of their lives like never before. When Josh did, he shed the blues. Today he's a much-admired schoolteacher and a meditator. When he talks about his time of depression, he now says, "I feel like I'm talking about someone else."

We don't mean to make this sound too easy. Embracing the idea that we should try turning inward to look at the one-minute mind takes time. It's just not our first impulse as human beings. There's an ancient Hindu story that captures this thought. The gods in the heavens, having watched man for many years, became annoyed by man's arrogance. They began plotting to punish him. In their wisdom, they decided the right punishment was to hide from man the truth about life. But where? One god suggested a hiding place at the top of the world's tallest mountain. "No," said the other gods, "too easy!" Another god suggested the bottom of the ocean. "No again," said the other gods, "still too easy!" After some thought the wisest god said, "Let's bury it deep within his own mind—he'll never think to look there!"

Of course, we do sometimes look inside for solutions to our stress. But we rarely seem to look there first, or often enough. We turn first to escapes like eating, watching TV, or shopping. And we turn too often to abusing drugs—including tobacco, alcohol, and caffeine. Yearning for these things isn't bad. It's normal. But we need to free ourselves from slavery to them. Compulsive behaviors of any kind are unsatisfactory attempts to relieve the distress created by the one-minute mind.

We can choose other ways that are more powerful. We all know that happiness does not come from money, possessions, power, or sex. As we age, we find that these are not so easy to come by anyway. They're not there for the plucking—and certainly not without stress. The more enduring rewards come from something we can learn to control: our selves and our minds.

Pen and Paper

Making Your Personal Escape List. How do you cope with stress and anxiety? On a piece of paper list as many one-minute escapes as you can—at least ten that you often indulge in. Now assess each one: Is it destructive or constructive? Mark each with a D or a C. Which ones might you rely on less? Which ones might you drop altogether?

3

The Drive for Peace

Your hearts know in silence the secrets of the days and the nights.

—KAHLIL GIBRAN

Finding Calm.   Take three deep breaths. Now, with your eyes closed, think of a recent time when you felt very relaxed. Repaint a picture of it in your mind. Was it at the seashore? In your garden? On a lake? In your favorite chair? Whatever the image, experience it again. Feel the air. Hear the sounds. Smell the scents. Settle into the tranquillity. If your mind strays, try to focus again on your image, and try to keep at it for one minute.

If you're like most people, you'll remember an image when your mind quieted and felt clear. You were mindful! You probably felt content. Why? You walked briefly out of the grasp of your one-minute mind. When you did, you felt the here and now. Not the past. Not the future. You felt happy in the moment—and you didn't tap a one-minute escape to get there.

Everyone feels a compulsion to revisit such moments. Let's call this "the drive for peace." Amid the busyness in your head—and amidst urges to eat, sleep, relate to others, make love—you feel a drive for calm. You may not feel it as strongly as hunger or lust. Still, it's with you always.

The drive for peace, if nurtured, can lift you directly into a pleasing, turmoil-free state of consciousness. This is a zone largely free of anxiety and stress. It's neither magical nor mythical. In fact, most people, by their twenties, have experienced such a pleasing state at least once. In studies, they report experiencing absolute peace and silence, being sunk in pleasant feelings, and losing a sense of time.

Odds are, you've tapped into this state of peace yourself. Maybe many times. Perhaps you've sensed it while in the woods, along the shore, at the crest of a mountain. Or maybe you felt it in moments of personal mastery—during a near-perfect golf swing, ski turn, tennis stroke, or basket-ball shot. You may even have sensed it in other people. If nothing else, recall the wide-eyed immersion of an infant in its new world. But so rare and fleeting are these moments that you have trouble describing them.

No matter what your own experience, in the pages that follow, you will learn that the drive lies within you. It may have arisen while you were at work, engaged in art, playing sports, at leisure, or immersed in prayer. What you've sensed on your own is that you don't have to look outside yourself to reduce your level of stress and anxiety. You can build on the powers you have already inside of yourself. You're just steps away from your own sense of "ahh!"

Many people repress their drive for inner peace for much of their lives. They think, "Someday, when I've finished raising a family and have retired, I will develop a state of satisfaction." They view the state of peace as always out ahead, in the future. They plan to tap the drive only after all of life's work is done. But this long-sighted view is really short-sighted. Enjoying the bounty of peaceful living starts with recognizing and nurturing the drive *today*—not tomorrow.

Random Acts of Peace

Sam Christy, sixty-seven, found the drive for peace within him. A retired technical illustrator, Sam has lived for a number of years by himself in a one-bedroom apartment. He says that he's never been happier or felt healthier. Still, his life's had both its ups and downs—like many of our lives. Sam could be like you, or like someone you know.

On the upside, Sam has liked his work. He's raised four kids. He's built a house. He's had a number of good, loyal friends. On the downside, he divorced his first wife when his kids were teenagers; his second wife divorced him when he was fifty-six. He fought through a two-year bout of depression when he was sixty-one. He had a heart attack when he was sixty-four.

Through it all, Sam still had those moments when he could just say, "ahh." In childhood, he found those moments at church, during prayer. "It was private, personal, peaceful," he says. "That's the place I'm looking for. That feeling is a very special place."

He recalls other moments as well. At work, he remembers when his drawings flowed effortlessly, when a picture he was rendering came out just right. He'd find that special peaceful place again.

When flying a small plane, Sam enjoyed the purr of the engine. And he relished smooth air. "There were certain times of day when the sun is down and it's hypnotic," he says. "It's smooth, it's silky." He felt an emotional, internal sense of peace.

Today, Sam finds the same place of peace in music. He puts on a CD of the passionate Italian operatic singer Andrea Bocelli. In one passage, Bocelli sings Giulio Caccini's aria, "Ave Maria." Sam becomes absorbed in Bocelli's breath and voice control. It transports him. "Music really touches me," he says.

In all these moments, Sam taps into his drive for peace. Simply put, he indulges his most human of impulses to find pleasure in the present moment. In this way, Sam shows what's possible for all of us. We can leave behind the pre-occupied one-minute mind. We can experience the place of peace first-hand. All we have to do is make the choice to do so.

A Natural Drive

Like Sam, you may have sensed this yearning for peace in many parts of your life. You, too, may think of it as a place of peace. You may be surprised to know, though, that the peaceful spot you find inside yourself is not unique. It probably resembles the place of peace found by many others. You probably experience it in the same way, too. That's because you have not stumbled onto something out of the ordinary. You've hit on something universal. The drive for peace is the yearning for tranquillity and the joy that accompanies it. It's part of the human experience.

Where does this universal drive come from? A pioneer in answering that question was famed psychologist Abraham Maslow. Maslow studied human experience for many years. He then outlined a theory, the "hierarchy of needs," that most people today take for granted. People strive first to satisfy bodily needs—air, water, food, sex, shelter. We next strive to satisfy basic needs—safety, love, respect, self-esteem, "belongingness." We go on striving to meet loftier needs—namely, how to live fulfilling lives.

Maslow showed that we follow a sort of escalating pleasure principle. After taking care of bodily business, we take care of mental business. We seek a very different kind of pleasure from each. But the motivation is the same: to improve our lives. We eat lunch to satiate hunger. We phone friends to affirm we belong. We change jobs to find more meaning. We "collect our thoughts" to reconnect with our place of peace. Although we may not think consciously about such choices, we do choose.

Maslow wrote, "Man demonstrates in his own nature a pressure toward fuller and fuller Being. . . in exactly the same naturalistic, scientific sense that an acorn may be said to be 'pressing toward' being an oak tree."

How do we describe what we're pressing toward? Usually we're not sure ourselves. But we know what feels right when we feel it. Or what washes away our worries. Or what brings us new perspectives and insights. Or what puts us in a pleasing groove. We discover through our own experience what researchers have revealed through experiments: *What makes all of our most pleasing moments most pleasing is absorption in the present moment.*

Average events during the day feel routine. They appear somewhat clear. They actively involve some of our mind. They reveal to us our ways of responding to the pleasure principle. But our state of mind as we tap the drive for peace isn't routine at all. The moments we experience are much clearer. They completely involve us in what we're doing. They bring us much closer to full focus—to a point where the mind is absorbed, yet aware.

Research by psychologist Gayle Privette shows that as we drive toward these golden moments of well-being we experience joy, freedom, unity, fulfillment, and awareness of power, among other qualities. In short, as we're absorbed in the present moment, we rise to a plateau of greater happiness. It's a plateau where our one-minute, escapist minds are hushed.

In such mindfulness we enjoy a pleasure of a much greater kind. It is the pleasure of experiencing the moment before our mind erupts into thought. Before the mind judges. Before it grasps. Before it fears. The mind simply soaks up the moment. Zen master Seung Sahn calls this, "the mind before thinking."

An Everyday Presence

A big misconception is that many of us are strangers to the drive for peace. This isn't so. If we're on the lookout, we find the drive in all we do. If you don't think so, reflect for a moment on one of the simpler pleasures of life: music. Remember a moment when you were swept up in one of your favorite melodies. Perhaps it was Brahms. Or Billie Holiday. Or Bruce Springsteen. Or Britney Spears. Or, as with Sam, Andrea Bocelli. Music often triggers a sense of well-being.

But the sweet sound of music is only one means to open ourselves to our most treasured internal drive. Of course, it doesn't work for everyone, either. Sara Atamian, thirty, had just given birth to her second child, a daughter. She was also working on her Ph.D. The twin tasks of mothering and research overwhelmed her. Worse, despite her accomplishments, she felt incomplete. She couldn't shake the feeling that her life was passing by her too quickly. "I felt like what I had achieved was not enough," she says.

Then, amid the pressures of life, Sara still found her place of peace. She hit upon it with the help of her new daughter. The first time she nursed the baby, Sara was looking outdoors. It was spring. A new leaf fell. The leaf twirled in the wind. It glinted in the sun. Her daughter nestled into her breast. All of a sudden, Sara experienced a special moment. It rose far above the mundane of many mothering tasks. It was peaceful, memorable.

Sara knew then that this was what she was searching for. "Being present in the moment was a revelation to me," she says. She recalls the image of nursing that day, now nine years ago, vividly. As for many people, Sara's moment of peace stays clear in her memory, even as other memories recede. The memory remains a guiding light for experiencing more of those moments.

Roy Babcock, sixty-one, was a runner for twenty-five years. He felt he had to run. "I had to run five days a week, or I would be a little crazy," he says. He ran one of six routes every day. Then he went to his teaching job at a prestigious law school. Funny thing about Roy's running, though. About three times a week he'd get home and he couldn't remember which of the routes he ran. "It's like I woke up," he says. "I'd been sleep-running."

Roy explains: After one to two miles, "I went on autopilot. It was a wonderful feeling I used to love about running." He'd become so absorbed with the feel of his body, the rhythm, the breathing, that the tireless workings of his mind took a time-out. Roy recalls the feeling as a "sense of self-forgetfulness." He prized those moments every day. Today he views them in the same way as Sara:

They are beacons for finding his way to a special place of peace.

Sara and Roy are special cases in some ways. They both reacted partly to the instincts of their bodies. Sara felt the natural soothing effect of mother touching child. Roy felt the calming of endorphins, the body's natural opiates, which are secreted during exercise. But something more was afoot. Sara and Roy were letting go. They were slipping into a tranquil refuge within themselves. This is a refuge that beckons to us always.

In so much of what we do, we face constant choices. In some of those choices, we listen to the voice of the one-minute mind. We fall prey to self-doubt, fear-mongering, or other unhealthy thought patterns. In other choices, we pay heed to the temptations of the one-minute escape. We become enslaved by distraction and addiction. But, in time, as we learn to listen to our minds and bodies, we hear more clearly the call of the third option, the drive for peace. The drive fights less fiercely for our attention than the hungry, escapist one-minute mind. But it takes us toward the sweetest points of life.

As we tune into the drive for peace, our appetite to indulge it grows. No surprise why. We feel healthier for it. Our gut calms down. Our sleep improves. Our stress dies back. Our anxiety quiets. Our sense of wholeness grows. By cultivating this peace of mind in the present moment, we nurture happiness in ourselves. The rest of this chapter describes where, within our lives, we already sense the drive for peace. It reaffirms that when we give ourselves over to the drive, we are opening ourselves to wonderful new possibilities.

Peace in Flow

Finding Flow.   Take three deep breaths. Now, again with your eyes closed, think of a recent time when you did something you enjoy. Playing golf. Arranging flowers. Bowling. Tying flies. Knitting. Playing chess. Skiing. Choose a time when you felt challenged, but skilled enough to match the challenge. In the same way you relived the last image, relive this one. Focus on this experience for one minute.

How does it feel? Different from visualizing a scene of peace? Somewhat different perhaps. But likely you felt similar sensations. Once again, you probably would like to experience more of these moments. You would like to feel your actions just "click." That's because you feel good when you're doing something well. And you far prefer such times to those when you just can't seem to get your act together.

The memory you've evoked is an example of *flow*. Psychologist Mihalyi Csikszentmihalyi, pioneer of the concept, first described flow after studying the satisfying experiences of artists, athletes, mountain climbers, and chess players. He later found that all kinds of people feel flow in all types of work and play—in everything from writing to conversation to science. Flow is important, because when you experience it, you truly enjoy life.

Csikszentmihalyi found that people in flow often report they know very clearly what they're doing moment to moment. They may have clear goals to guide them. They also get immediate feedback—the score of a game, the sound of a melody. And they feel that their ability matches the opportunity for action. This is one of the main principles of flow: The better you match your skills to the challenges of life, the more you'll enjoy yourself.

Csikszentmihalyi and Giovanni Moneta, of Finland's Institute of Occupational Health, showed how important this is in a complex experiment. They equipped two hundred Chicago high-schoolers with pagers. Eight times a day, at a random radio signal, the fourteen- to seventeen-year-olds filled out a two-minute questionnaire. They recorded what they were doing and how they felt. The results? Polled at random at school, with family, with friends, and in solitude, the adolescents revealed they felt happiest in all cases when skills and challenges were balanced.

Why is this so? Look at it this way: If you think your skills fall short, you feel anxiety. If you think your skills go over the top, you get bored. You feel great only when your skills and challenges are more equal. When the balance gets out of whack, so does your sense of well-being.

Searching for flow, people naturally try to improve their skills. They adhere to a sort of Goldilocks principle: Take the porridge of life not too hot (too challenging, making us anxious), nor too cold (too easy, leaving us bored), but just right. Most of us get pretty good at this Goldilocks balancing process. Although two out of ten people say they've never felt flow, the same number say they feel it several times a day.

When we're in flow, we feel great. We think, "This is what I'm living for!" If you're strumming a guitar, volleying a tennis ball, hitting a golf ball, rolling a bowling ball, pitching a horseshoe, you do best when you're in flow. Notice the key characteristic of flow: When you experience it, you enter a state of absorption. In other words, you are following the lead of your drive for peace.

What are other elements of flow? Csikszentmihalyi confirms that when you're in flow, your attention is intensely concentrated. Your mind excludes unimportant content. You find flow rewarding for its own sake. He also says that you lose your self-consciousness. "Being able to forget temporarily who we are," he notes, "seems to be very enjoyable."

So when you experience flow in, say, a game, you're losing yourself in it. Your one-minute mind quiets. Your thought-filled one-minute escapes evaporate. You operate on instinct. You are totally mindful of your action, not your thought. You may even perform better. Perhaps that's why Yogi Berra said, "You can't think and hit at the same time."

Let's be clear: When you're tapping the drive for peace—and experiencing the peaceful mind disengaged from the engine of thought—you don't lose your thinking ability. You just leave aside the one-minute mind. Stress and anxiety then slip out of the picture. You are mindful! And you resolve to come back to this state more often. This is a universal instinct. You can use it to access your place of peace at will.

Peace in Peak Performance

Many people tap the drive for peace during what sports psychologists call "peak performance." At its simplest, peak performance is performing beyond your normal capacity. It's optimal functioning—when everything goes right. Like most people, you probably experience peak performance more rarely than flow. But during such performances, you've another chance to catch a glimpse of the place of peace within yourself. This is the place where the one-minute mind shuts down and the focused mind appears.

Dot Smerciak, the sixty-one-year-old nursing supervisor from Chapter 1, remembers the pleasure of peak performance. Until her early fifties, Dot played tournament volleyball. Dot and her team were good. She remembers the feeling of a great game, and a great win. "You get in an intense game, and all of your worries are washed away," she says.

That was particularly true when her team was trying to qualify for national competition. She was in an evening tournament, and her team was playing nonstop from 9 P.M. to 1 A.M. In a best-of-five match, her team lost the first two games, and was down 11–4 in the third. In a wild reversal, her team rallied to win 15–11, and then won the next two games. "As exhausted as I was, I had this feeling of total euphoria," she says. "Boy, we really gave of ourselves."

Dot and her teammates had stretched themselves to summon their peak skills. And they had met the toughest of challenges. That evening of intense concentration remains a vivid memory for Dot to this day, years later. In some ways, Dot had set herself up to tap the drive for peace. In that way, she's like many athletes. As she says, "Anyone who has given themselves very intensely knows that. . . you get that feeling of euphoria and well-being."

Research shows that peak-performance feelings are much the same in all people, no matter what the sport or activity. With peak performance comes absorption, focus, full attention, spontaneous action and thought. Notice how similar the characteristics of peak performance are to flow. Both introduce people to a means of eliminating the one-minute mind. And both take us to a place that feels timeless, joy-filled, and deeply satisfying.

Peak performance in sports may come easier to professionals. Some pros feel that tapping the drive for peace rates as the biggest reward of sport. So says Phil Jackson, the revered basketball coach. "What drives most basketball players is not the money or the adulation, but their love of the game," he says in his autobiography. "They live for those moments when they can lose themselves completely in the action and experience the pure joy of competition."

Jackson worked for nine years as the coach of the Chicago Bulls. He led such larger-than-life players as Michael Jordan and Scottie Pippen to six National Basketball Association championships. When Jordan retired, Jackson moved to the Los Angeles Lakers. There he led players like Shaquille O'Neal and Kobe Bryant to play extraordinary basketball and win their first NBA championship in twelve years. Through it all, Jackson has insisted on a coaching style that revolves around alertness.

"The secret is not thinking," he says. "That doesn't mean being stupid; it means quieting the endless jabbering of thoughts so that your body can do instinctively what it's been trained to do without the mind getting in the way."

The drive for peace is simply that—an instinct for living without the mind getting in the way. Jackson taught this as a principle to get his teams to play the best basketball they could. Some players call this concept developing the "cocoon of concentration"—total alertness on the floor.

"All of us have had flashes of this sense of oneness— making love, creating a work of art—when we're completely immersed in the moment, inseparable from what we're doing," says Jackson. "This kind of experience happens all the time on the basketball floor; that's why the game is so intoxicating."

As in basketball, so in life. Joy comes from pure concentration on the present moment. In mindfulness. In tapping the drive for peace. But note that studies show that peak performance is common outside of sports, too. Some people experience such peaks while engaged in art, in personal relationships, in struggles against death, or in intellectual pursuits. So you may have tasted the drive in peak performances of your own.

Once again, you see that the drive for peace is within you. You have the power to cultivate it. You have the good fortune to find your special place through it. The drive runs throughout human experience. Tapping it is as human as longing for a relationship with another human being. For many people, tapping the drive is irresistible.

Peace in Peak Experience

Losing Yourself. Think again of the vision you evoked at the start of the chapter. Now, as you close your eyes, trace the image back to an earlier, stronger experience of the same sense of well-being. Scan all the way back to childhood. Spend some time raising the image from your memory. Once again, fix it in your mind. Feel the feeling. Sense the sensations. Stay with this for a minute.

Were you able to summon a stronger image? Could you recapture the original feeling? If you're like most people, you will have experienced at least once an episode far stronger than either flow or peak performance. Most people have experienced a state of consciousness where they felt more than absorption and full attention. They felt peace, joy, and an "understanding of the universe." This is what we're talking about. This is called a "peak experience."

Peak experiences can happen at any time, anywhere. A good example comes from the experience of Billie Jean King. In the 1960s and 1970s, King became the most successful woman athlete of all time. She won twenty Wimbledon tennis titles. People know her best for beating Bobby Riggs in the 1973 "Battle of the Sexes" in tennis. She had extraordinary drive.

In the mid-1970s, King's career hit its top, and she wrote in her autobiography what it was like to hit a perfect shot: "They don't come along very often, but when they do, they're great. It gives me a marvelous feeling of almost perfect joy."

She then explained: "My concentration is so perfect it almost seems as though I'm able to transport myself beyond the turmoil on the court to some place of total peace and calm. . . . My heart pounds, my eyes get damp, and my ears feel like they're wiggling, but it's also just totally peaceful. It's almost like having an orgasm—it's exactly like that. And when it happens I want to stop the match and grab the microphone and shout, '*That's* what it's all about.'"

Abraham Maslow coined the term "peak experience." And some of Maslow's most famous work came from studying hundreds of people who had peak experiences. As with people in flow and during peak performance, Maslow found that those in peak experience felt absorption, joy, awareness. But they encountered something much richer, too. They often felt their sense of self merge with the world around them. They felt less judgmental, more complete, more compassionate. They felt the unity of all things. And they felt fear and anxiety vanish.

From his studies, Maslow sketched the "identity" of people in peak experience. He said they feel at the peak of their powers, "in the groove," free of blocks, inhibitions, cautions, doubts. They feel free of the past and future, more in the present. They feel more creative, sometimes poetic, often playful and good-humored. They don't feel they're fighting as much with themselves. They're more at peace.

The peak experience, though intense and infrequent, appears to be another way people tap into the drive for peace. Unlike the experience of flow and peak performance, you can't exactly set yourself up for a peak experience. Peak experiences generally just happen. And they can happen in any line of work or play.

No surprise that one of the geniuses of the twentieth century wrote of what appears to have been intellectual peak experiences. Albert Einstein revealed his experiences in a letter to one of his old friends, Queen Elizabeth of Belgium. It was January 1939. His work went well, Einstein said. But he was haunted by the unfolding tragedy in Hitler's Germany. He wrote:

> Still, there are moments when one feels free from one's own identification with human limitation and inadequacies. At such moments, one imagines that one stands on some spot of a small planet, gazing in amazement at the cold yet profoundly moving beauty of the eternal, the unfathomable; life and death flow into one, and there is neither evolution nor destiny; only being.

You certainly don't have to be a star sports figure or a genius to enjoy a peak experience, though. Recent research suggests that more than three quarters of all people have had peak experiences. Many people even have them as kids, before the age of fourteen. When you do have one, it remains a vivid memory.

What triggers peak experiences? Nature, sex, music, sport, or art, among other things. In one study of artists, moments of creativity and beauty triggered the greatest number of peak experiences. The artists characterized their peak experiences in the same way as people from all other walks of life. They cherished the joy and fulfillment, meaning and personal value, intensity and absorption.

The picture that emerges is clear: Peak experiences are another way that we tap into the drive for peace. They may be rare in our lives, but the potential to experience them lies imbedded within us. They turn out to be one of the most meaningful of human experiences.

British poet Alfred Lord Tennyson wrote of his own spontaneous peak experiences:

> All at once, as it were out of the intensity of the consciousness of individuality, the individuality itself seemed to dissolve and fade away into boundless being, and this not a confused state, but the clearest of the clearest, the surest of the surest. . . utterly beyond words.

Peaks in Religion

What is the ultimate experience in the drive for peace? For some people, it is a peak of spiritual or religious realization. Over the millennia, millions have experienced such moments, not just the saints and prophets. So commonly do people report them that we have to consider them part of normal human experience.

In one survey, roughly a third of Americans agreed with the statement: "You felt as though you were very close to a powerful spiritual force that seemed to lift you out of your self." Some of these people said they had felt that way often or several times. These religious or spiritual incidents generally last less than half an hour, often just a few minutes or less.

Stories of spiritual peaks fill the pages of religious history. They appear commonly in Muslim, Jewish, and Christian texts. One of the renowned stories in Christianity is of Saint Teresa of Ávila. Raised in a family of twelve children, in 1535 Teresa de Cepeda y Ahumada ran away from her home in the Castilian town of Ávila. She became a nun. Over her lifetime, Teresa experienced and described a five-part ladder of prayer. The ladder detailed a path to religious advancement. It called for prayer with growing concentration at each level. The ladder peaked with union with God. In this state, one is "wholly absorbed in God's indescribable greatness," Saint Teresa said. "There is no feeling, but only rejoicing, unaccompanied by any understanding of the thing in which the soul is rejoicing."

In this state, Teresa became absorbed entirely in unity. "There is a self-forgetfulness which is so complete that it really seems as though the soul no longer existed," she said.

Saint Teresa and other figures had the ability to lift themselves into a place of peace that was extraordinary. But in some ways, religious figures were climbing the same mountain as the rest of us today. They just happened to get beyond the foothills and close to the summit. They did not plan these events, any more than people today can plan spiritual peaks. But they consciously opened themselves to the drive for peace through prayer, contemplation, solitude, and other techniques.

One historical figure tells an unusual tale about his religious peaks. Composer Johannes Brahms could call forth such peaks almost at will. "It has always been such a wonderful experience," he said in an 1896 interview, when he was sixty-three. "I felt that I was, for the moment, in tune with the Infinite, and there is no thrill like it." He then revealed how this worked. Before starting to compose, he contemplated the thought in John 10:30, when Jesus said: "I and my Father are one." Brahms said this awakened the sense of unity within himself. He could then lift himself to a very special place. Brahms said of these rare, inspired moods:

> I immediately feel vibrations. . . . In this exalted state, I see clearly what is obscure in my ordinary moods. . . . Those vibrations assume the forms of distinct mental images. . . . Straightaway the ideas flow in upon me, directly from God, and not only do I see distinct themes in my mind's eye, but they are clothed in the right forms, harmonies and orchestration. Measure by measure, the finished product is revealed to me.

Brahms claimed that all great composers and poets— Milton, Tennyson, Wordsworth, Mozart, Beethoven— strove to tap into this same power. He even suggested that anyone can tap this power, and that Jesus himself made this clear. "We can appropriate it for our own upbuilding right here and now," Brahms said. "Jesus Himself is very explicit about this, saying, 'Ask and it shall be given you, seek and ye shall find; knock and it shall be opened unto you.'"

Brahms was exceptional. He demonstrated a rare experience, as Jesus said, that "the kingdom of Heaven is within you." But you may have also felt hints of what Brahms describes. If so, you've seen first-hand the drive to seek a special place of peace. You're likely to agree that whether in flow, peak performance, peak experience, or religious peaks, the instinct to find the place of peace typifies human strivings of all kinds.

A Quality Drive

Across a range of human experience, we find the same thing: We can find peace, and the path to peace, within ourselves. You have already tasted at least hints of a stress-free place. It might be in daily life. It might be in engaging work. It might be in sports. It might be in spiritual realization. But in all cases, the capacity and drive to experience it is within ourselves. We know it in our hearts.

What is the mind like as it advances into the stress-free zone on the path to peace? At its most basic, it's a mind aware, absorbed, concentrated, joyful. It's a mind freed from bondage to mental chattering and heckling. It's a mind no longer thirsting for the one-minute escape. Disengaged from habitual one-minute thinking, it is a mind that charms, liberates, and draws us irresistibly.

The fact is, you have the capacity to learn to be aware—mindful—of your surroundings before you think about them. What gets you into trouble is the endless thinking and feeling triggered by mental habits of the one-minute mind. The thinking buries you in a pile of stressful and anxiety-producing thought. The sad fact is that you've trained your mind to work that way. Trained it so well that it now has a mind of its own. The result can sometimes be tragic—

as when panic attacks or heart disease impair your health in middle age.

But you can also train your mind to go in another direction. You can nudge it toward the drive for peace. This is true no matter what your work, age, faith, goals, mental capacity, state of health, or hobbies or sports interests. To be sure, you can hope and wait for rare spontaneous moments. But you have an appealing alternative: Close the door on the one-minute mind—and learn to access a place of peace and joy directly. You do this through the practice of meditation, the topic of the next chapter.

Pen and Paper

Taking Stock of Peace.   List the hours of the day down the side of a piece of paper, the way they would appear in an appointment book. For each hour of the day, mark in an element of everyday awareness, flow, peak performance, or peak experience that you may have experienced. These are your past appointments with the drive for peace. You can see they're already a part of the fabric of your life. Now you're ready to strengthen them.

4
One-Minute Meditation

Don't just do something, sit there!

—Unknown

When Paul Neary turned sixty-six, he began to ease into retirement by coming to the office every day a bit later than usual. The problem was, he no longer got a parking space a few steps from the door. He had to park in the boonies. "It used to make me angry," he says. No matter that the path to his office crossed a serene hilltop carpeted with lush grass and graced with stately shade trees.

Paul stayed angry for days until he realized he had a choice—"a good surprise" he calls it. The minute or so walk to the office door could remain an irritant. He could let it bring to a boil every morning his sense of indignation. Or he could view it as an opportunity to relieve stress through meditation.

Naturally, when he saw he was missing a chance to defuse discontent, he chose option two. He focused fully on his breath and footsteps each day as he made his way across the asphalt and through the doors. In the one minute of walking from his car to the office, Paul sampled the benefits of meditation that he had enjoyed in longer increments of time for more than twenty years. "It's always given me peace of mind," he says.

Now seventy, Paul conveys the message of this book: You can take any minute in life and turn it into a minute of better living. As some Japanese meditators say, you can "steal moments" from the day. Every minute you lapse into mindlessness offers a chance to tap instead the drive for peace. "You think it's a waste, but it's not," says Paul. "You give dignity to the shortness of time."

By trying each one-minute exercise in the last three chapters, you have learned a number of meditative skills. In this chapter, you'll learn how to meditate more formally— to "sit." With step-by-step instructions, you will find you can enjoy not just a minute, but five or ten, or twenty minutes. And you'll begin to see meditation as a journey—in both self-control and self-development.

You took the first step in learning to meditate in Chapter 1. There, you sampled meditation as a refuge from stress and anxiety. You learned that mental traffic in the one-minute mind creates stress. And stress may lead to muscle tension, headaches, high blood pressure, heart disease, depression, and anxiety disorders.

You took a second step in Chapter 2. There you sampled meditation to understand your impulses to quell stress with half measures. You learned that we scan constantly for escapes. Some escapes, like exercise, are healthy. Some, like distraction and addiction, are not.

You took a third step in Chapter 3. There you sampled meditation to awaken the drive for peace within yourself. You learned that you have probably visited the special place of peace already. But you came at it *indirectly*—in art, sports, nature, love, music, prayer, and everyday life.

In this chapter, you'll take a fourth step. Here you'll learn to acquire the mental tools to deal with stress on your own, and in depth—whether crossing a parking lot or sitting on a cushion, driving your car or making love to your partner or spouse. You'll learn that you can find content-ment by tapping into your drive for peace *directly*.

The Practice of Peace

There are only a few prerequisites for meditation: the intention to sit still, quiet, alert, aware of the present moment. The desire to develop a capacity to just "be" rather than the compulsion to always "do." The commit-ment to be mindful and to attain the state that allows release from the ruthless grip of the one-minute mind. With that attitude, the basic practice is simple:

1. Sit comfortably in a quiet place.
2. Place your hands in your lap, one hand over the other.
3. Close your eyes.
4. Breathe deeply two or three times. Inhale fully. Exhale fully.
5. Release the tension in your face, jaw, neck, and shoulders.
6. Feel your in-breath and out-breath. Let them take their natural pace, as your body requires.
7. Concentrate all your attention on these breaths. Feel the air flow through your nostrils. Feel the rise and fall of your belly.
8. Acknowledge emerging thoughts, sensations, feelings, and images. Let them go and focus again on your breathing.
9. Continue for one to ten minutes. Just breathing!

That's it! Those are the basics of "sitting." You now have the know-how to beat the dissatisfaction that plagues peo-ple the world over—the plague of the one-minute mind.

Although the one-minute mind seems to defy change, you *can* change it. You can concentrate it. You can steady it. You can be mindful of it. Right now!

Of course, reading about a skill is a lot easier than mastering it. But the more you practice, the better you'll get. The quality of your attention from minute to minute sharpens the quality of your attention day to day, year to year, and ultimately throughout life. You'll find it easier and easier to swing into the groove of contentment.

What do most people say about that groove? A study of almost 1,000 people gives a good sample. Each person, who regularly practiced some kind of relaxation technique, was asked to cite words that typified his or her experience. Ten words summarized the effect of massage, muscle relaxation, yoga stretching, breathing, imagery, and meditation. The words were "joyful," "distant," "calm," "aware," "prayerful," "accepted," "untroubled," "limp," "silent," "mystery." But just four words captured the effect of meditation: "calm," "aware," "joyful," and "prayerful."

Some of these effects come with much practice, ten, twenty, or thirty minutes a day. But you can ease yourself into sitting by meditating in shorter snatches. Just one minute helps reposition your intention from mindlessness to mindfulness. In that time, you can start to turn your back on the hot zone of scattered thinking and face the cool zone of focused concentration. You can summon your resolve. Find your breath. Witness the mental chatter. And momentarily sense the possibility of tranquillity.

Your Practice in Action

You may be a bit like Paul Neary when he started meditating twenty years ago. You may have second thoughts about trying something so foreign to the American mind as sitting and doing nothing. "I'm an anxious person," Paul admits. "At the beginning, I was a little bit afraid of meditation." Some fear and doubt is natural. After all, cartoonists have lampooned meditation for years. They've made monks on mountaintops the butt of jokes. They imply that, in sitting, you drain personality from your life. And who wants to go flat like an old soda?

But meditation doesn't dull your wit. It doesn't ruin your taste for life. It doesn't sap your creativity or energy. It simply enhances every moment with newfound clarity. It injects into the flow and chaos of life a measure of cool-headedness. "It has enriched my life," says Paul, who started sitting in his forties.

To be sure, many people try meditation just to cut stress. That's why Paul has always found time to sit, whether for an hour or ten minutes. He even finds meditation cuts stress in small emergencies. He tells a story to make his point. On a plane flight three years ago, he quaked with his lifelong fear of landing. As the plane descended, a novel notion hit him: "I said to myself when the plane began to shake, 'Why don't you meditate?'" So he counted his in-breaths and out-breaths. And in five to ten minutes, "the anxiety went away," he says.

But meditation teaches you about more than calming your nerves. Reflecting on life, Paul notes how he fell into a trap many of us do: He ruminated over his past. He fretted about what he could have done better. He dwelled on his shortcomings as a physician and father. But meditation helped him be more accepting of himself. It made him more cognizant of his accomplishments. "It changes one's outlook on things," he says, "You forget the past; it cannot be changed."

As you taste the fruits of meditation, you may want to deepen your practice, like Paul. If so, you can start sitting once or twice daily for ten minutes or more. The longer sits give you a grip on mindfulness that carries over into the shorter ones. As you meditate in longer stretches, you'll want to pay attention to meditation's finer points:

Posture

You can sit on a chair, a cushion, the edge of a bed, or a couch. But sit erect. Lift the top of your head toward the ceiling. Keep your chin in, chest out, buttocks back. Let your body hang from your frame. Sit with your knees lower than your thighs, if you can. That way, you can keep your spine straighter with less effort. Remember, the object is to stay relaxed but alert. The right posture helps generate an alert, focused mind.

Breathing

Most people breathe in one of two ways: with their chest or belly. Belly breathing, though not glamorous at the beach, is more natural. When you were a baby, you always breathed with your belly (because your ribs were too flexible to do anything else). Belly breathing works this way: As you take a breath, the layer of muscle below your lungs, called the diaphragm, contracts to draw in air. Your tummy pushes out. Chest breathing works differently. You chest breathe by expanding your rib cage. Breathing with your chest suggests you are tense. You tend to breathe fast and shallow. Your tummy hardly moves.

To learn the difference, place one hand on your belly and the other on your chest. Now look down at your hands.

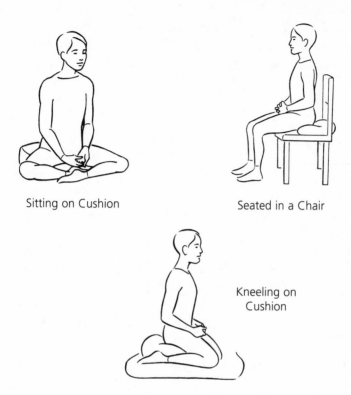

Sitting on Cushion

Seated in a Chair

Kneeling on Cushion

See if you can keep the upper hand still while the lower one moves with the breath. When you sit, you should seek the same movement. Let your belly relax. Draw longer, deeper breaths into your lungs. You'll find that this kind of breathing induces calm like no other single technique.

Focus Point

What do you concentrate on when you're breathing? Most often, you should choose the most prominent sensation. This may be the feel of air flowing in and out of your nose, cool going in, warm going out. Or it may be the rise and fall of your belly. See for yourself which works best. As you get more experienced, you may switch from one to the other to refresh your focus.

Muscles

The first indicator of a relaxing mind is relaxing muscles. So after relaxing your face and shoulders, if you feel tense, relax each of the muscles in your body. Start with your face and move down your torso and out each limb. Among the most sensitive muscles to the one-minute mind are the jaw, tongue, and vocal chords. They often shadow your internal dialogue. Try to relax all three. Check on them often. When they relax, you'll find you've shifted to belly breathing, and your thoughts have quieted down.

Counting

If you have trouble following your breaths, count them, one to ten, or one to five. Count both the in-breath and out-breath, or count just out-breaths. Do whatever helps you maintain your thread of attention. You can also count in declining sequence, one to five, one to four, one to three, one to two, one to one. You may also say to yourself "in" on the in-breath, "out" on the out-breath. Let your body breathe naturally. Try not to breathe like it's your job.

Timing

You can practice for just one minute, but if possible, mix short sits with longer ones. There isn't any "right" amount of meditation. But research shows that sitting for up to fifteen minutes every day appears to be very effective. More seems to have added benefit. In any case, the skill of meditation is not different from the skills of ballet, or skateboarding, or guitar. You get out of it what you put in.

As for when you sit, work it into the day whenever you can regularly find a quiet, free moment. It can be any time from when you get up to when you go to bed. A lot of people prefer early morning and early evening. Many teachers advise against meditating right after a meal, because you may get sleepy. But it's better to pause whenever you have a chance than not to pause at all.

A Sense of Place

You can practice anywhere, anytime. But when you're sitting formally, try to find a spot where you can sit every day. If you can, go somewhere that puts you in the mood. Some people make an altar, a place for only meditation and prayer. You may have no choice but to listen to the comings and goings of your family. You may hear them getting up. You may smell popcorn from the microwave after school. Ask friends and family not to interrupt you, and turn the phone off.

What Can You Expect?

Many people find they take to meditation immediately. The first time they sit, they feel calmer within minutes. Recall forty-year-old Kevin Nuñez from Chapter 1. Kevin had become angry with his wife. He fumed over her on-line chat with other men. In an effort to calm himself, he tried sitting quietly, aware. He focused first on the sounds outside his home, then the appearance of the room, then the feel of his body, and then awareness of his thoughts.

The very first time he tried to meditate, Kevin got up about thirty minutes early in the morning, before his four children or wife. He sat in a chair and drew up straight—"like a king in a throne," he says. He sat for a bit less than ten minutes. "It was incredibly peaceful," he remembers. "I'm not a morning person, and getting up early, before everyone, was special. I felt very refreshed and relaxed, almost like I'd stayed in bed that extra half hour."

We hear this sort of story all the time. Some people find the calm in meditation right away. But not everyone finds the first sit so refreshing. Maria Borne says she could sit only three and a half minutes the first time. She tried to follow her breath, but she couldn't. This frustrated her. So she just forced herself. "It took a couple of sittings to learn to let go" of mental chatter and pent-up tension, she says.

Others find something in between. Recall Craig Moser, the student, athlete, and fraternity president from Chapters 1 and 2. Craig, who often drank to quell stress, meditated for the first time during a classroom talk on the subject. He sat still on the floor, counting his breaths, for ten minutes.

"It was a very new thing for me and was very calming," he says. But what he most felt was "real physical tiredness" and even sleepiness from working fourteen to eighteen hours a day. "I was able to see the consequences of my lifestyle."

No matter what your first experience—whether you *feel* great or not—know that you *are* making headway. This became clear after some pioneering research by physician Herbert Benson at Harvard Medical School in the 1970s. Benson showed that meditation flips a sort of physiologic switch in your mind and body. It turns on the "relaxation response." This response triggers changes that are opposite those of the fight-or-flight response.

During the relaxation response, your body uses less oxygen. Your breathing and heart rate slow. In Benson's initial study of experienced meditators, heart rate declined by three beats per minute during meditation. Oxygen consumption fell 10 to 20 percent in three minutes. To repeat, Benson found that no matter whether you *feel* you're doing a good job meditating, these changes still take place, even for beginners. In experienced meditators, they begin in as little as two minutes.

Benson first tested people doing Transcendental Meditation (see Chapter 6). But Benson soon found similar results for other varieties of meditation. So long as you follow the basic steps we've outlined above, you will experience the same effect. Benson and his team concluded that two steps during sitting were pivotal. The first: focusing on a repetitive word, sound, prayer, phrase, image, or action like breathing. The second: passively returning to that focus after each mental side trip.

The practice of meditation sounds too simple to be true. But note the nature of the challenge. You're marrying an uncommon couple: relaxation and awareness. *You are developing the skill to stay fully relaxed while fully alert.*

You can now answer a question most people ask: "How does meditation differ from sleep?" The answer is simple: In meditation, you stay fully awake even while you enter a state of deep rest, and you enter that state in a matter of minutes. When you sleep, your oxygen consumption declines only 8 percent (half as much as meditation), and only after four to five hours.

Dropping so quickly into a restful state is what many people like most about sitting. Consider Maria Borne once again. Maria now works in a civilian office. She has a new routine. After spending four hours on the phone in her job, she goes home for lunch. She then sits for 20 minutes before returning to work. "It's like I'm starting the day all over again," she says. "It's like taking a nap but you're not asleep. You can kind of get two days in one."

The best part about rest from meditation is that it has a carryover effect. The calm of sitting helps you stay calm later. Research even reveals why the relaxation response throttles down your reaction to norepinephrine. When you are frightened, your body still doses you with this stimulant. And normally it would incite pangs of stress and anxiety. But with a regular sitting practice, your heart rate and blood pressure simply don't jump so easily.

The Practice of Mindfulness

Seeing the Waterfall.   Take three deep, cleansing breaths. Now watch for a thought to form in your mind. Follow the cascade of thoughts that follow. Can you distinguish how one links to the next? You probably will have trouble. But notice something about this "mental noting," as it's called: You're using your mind to observe itself. Keep on for a minute and mentally label the thoughts popping from your brain.

If meditation helped lick stress only by calming your body, that alone would make the practice worth your time. But if you keep at it, you will find that calming is just an early milestone. The more you practice meditation, the farther you can go. What you see along the road—what you observe—makes you more skilled in handling stress, anxiety, and other life challenges.

One way to think about meditation is that it helps you strengthen two skills. The first is concentration. By repeatedly bringing your focus back to your breath, you build your mental muscle to focus narrowly. The second is staying mindful. By repeatedly acknowledging, moment to moment, all the goings-on in your mind, you build your mental muscle to stay aware of everything in the present moment.

The skill of concentration, to oversimplify a bit, calms your mind. When you concentrate, you can decrease stress by triggering the relaxation response. The skill of mindfulness, to simplify as well, acts as a more powerful therapy. It opens your eyes to the workings of your mind, and thus helps to keep you from getting stressed to begin with.

Why is this so? Remember, at any moment, your mind is loaded with thoughts, emotions, sensations, images, memories, and so on. As each arises, you typically react to it. When the force of one thought strikes your mind, you typically launch an opposing force. You can't help yourself. You've learned from childhood to hit back. Launching an inner conflict may even become a reflex. You may have sensed the reacting mind in the meditation above.

We've also learned that the mind runs down a lot of repetitive tracks. If you see something, you judge it (good, bad, or neutral). If you taste something, you grasp it (grasp for more if it's good, less if bad). If you feel something, you react with a measure of fear (fear of losing what's good or facing more if bad). You may then catastrophize, joyride, go overboard, or succumb to other traps. And the destination of following such mindless tracks is the land of stress, stress, and more stress.

But seeing is believing. That's the principal of mindfulness. When you see something for what it is, you can change it. With knowledge, you are empowered. That's why meditation can help you deal with the causes of stress. You don't learn about causes from someone else, or just from a book. You must look for the causes yourself. You must experience the sights and sounds of your mind on your own. And as a variation of the old adage goes, by seeing the problem yourself, you're halfway to the solution.

In practicing mindfulness, you become your own mental auditor. As if with clipboard in hand, you record the junkets of the one-minute mind. You soon see patterns in where the mind is going. With a clear picture of how the mind travels, you change your perspective on things. You can't help but become less reflexive, less critical. That's because you've become wiser about yourself. So you react less out of habit, and less inappropriately. You respond more, and more thoughtfully. You take control of your life, because you are taking control of your mind.

Deepening Mindfulness

When we talk about staying mindful, we are, in a way, suggesting you work with two parts of your mind: the part that acts and the part that witnesses the action. The acting part is the busy mind. The witnessing part is the observer. The acting part rushes around on the field of play. The witnessing part, above the fray, sits in the stands and gapes at the volley of thought and emotion. Like a spectator, the witnessing part sees first-hand that the one-minute mind is running a complex game.

Your challenge as a witness is twofold. First, of course, is to watch your breathing. Second, to acknowledge the endless wanderings of the one-minute mind.

When you notice a thought, silently say, "thinking" and go back to your breath. If you see an image, say, "seeing." If you feel an itch, "itching." If you feel hungry, "hunger." Keep an attitude of friendly acceptance. Don't try to stop your thinking. Or quiet your emotions. Or numb your senses. You can never do that. Just try to stay fully aware of the flow of thoughts and images in your head. Observe the wanderings with a sense of wonder and detachment. Then you go back to breathing.

The process of reforming the mind is like breaking a dog of car chasing. Many dogs, like minds, just can't help themselves. They go after every car passing on the street. How silly! It's just a steady stream of Chevys, Fords, and Hondas going by. The cars come into view one moment, and leave the next. Dogs don't need to bark at each one or sniff the occupants. And you don't need to focus on this mental "traffic" either. This traffic is like the flow of thought in the one-minute mind. Through training, we can teach dogs, and our minds, to watch traffic without actively chasing after it.

Remember that meditation is not introspection. That may seem hard to believe at first. Your mind is so clever at outwitting your mental forces of focus that you seem to be inspecting your interior all the time. You tell yourself over and over that your job is to just breathe mindfully. Nothing else! But in reality you have a hard time staying on task. You end up thinking all the time. Remember, you're not setting out to analyze and think things through. You're setting out just to observe. Your role: to stay totally aware of—yet free of interest in—everything about yourself.

Some people think that when you find your mind wandering, you're not meditating. A failure of focus is a failure of your sitting practice. But far from being a failure of meditation, noticing your thoughts *is* meditation.

You may feel split, though. One moment you're aware of your breath. The next you're observing your thoughts. How do you stay mindful of both? Take heart. With practice, you will get better at going in both directions: focusing on your breath and noting your thoughts. In doing so, you will be building a key mental muscle. A muscle that helps you follow the mind wherever it goes. And when you condition this mental muscle, a wonderful thing happens. You fall victim to the one-minute mind less often. You struggle less with the bad feeling the one-minute mind can unleash. And you less often feel robbed of your mind's potential for peace.

Through this whole process, remain gentle with yourself. Don't get angry at the ramblings of your mind. Don't blame yourself for lack of progress. Befriend your mind. As you get better, you'll feel like you're holding up a mirror to the present moment. As you follow the action scene by scene, detail by detail, you will get a clearer understanding of what is there. Don't judge. Don't condemn. Don't repress. See the moment, as some meditation teachers say, with "choiceless awareness."

The result will be that you won't get so jumpy over trifles. You'll react less, and less quickly. You'll let things flow, and you'll realize: "That's where my anger comes from." "That's why I feel such stress." "That's why I'm anxious." With this awareness comes insight, acceptance, and compassion for yourself and others.

Mindfulness in Action

Kevin Nuñez is a good example of how mindfulness meditation works in real life. A meditator for three years, Kevin did us a big favor. He interrupted two of his sits expressly to take written notes on his mental wanderings. His notes offer a mirror for all of us to see what goes on even in the mind of someone who has begun a serious sitting practice. They show how the mind fills easily with the creative and mundane, the constructive and destructive.

In Kevin's case, the mundane came first. He noted his thoughts of reminding himself to write down his thoughts. He also noted thinking that his kids, goofing off and disturbing his sit, were probably too rowdy and spoiled. You may have had similar run-of-the-mill thoughts in the first moments of sitting down to meditate.

After ten minutes, Kevin relaxed. His mind then poured forth thoughts in movie-like form. These probably emerged partly from his unconscious. In one image, he was driving. As he pulled out of his son's junior high school, a 1960s-vintage car rammed him. He felt twinges of stress. Then another image arose. He thought about when his son was a five-year-old (a memory of a long-ago past). His son was running with other kids in the street. Again Kevin felt a twinge of stress, as he worried over his son's safety.

In simply noting such thoughts, Kevin could quickly learn his mind's habits. Some of his habits clearly would provoke stress. Others are not harmful. In his second sitting, Kevin again slipped into deep meditation. One image he stopped to note: He was in a rocky desert, as in Saudi Arabia. He was a member of a Bedouin clan. As camels milled around, he ate campfire fare for dinner. His chief concern: "How do I go to the bathroom with this Bedouin robe on?"

An odd thought! Where did it come from? Kevin doesn't know. But all of our minds raise this kind of whimsical traffic. This isn't unusual. But sitting helps you see it. It helps you see that you can just let a lot of it go by. You don't have to stop and struggle with it. Cars come and cars go. They are the creativity of the mind working. They may have nothing to do with your enduring self. You just don't need to deal with them.

Of course, some traffic comes from worries that are real. But even then, meditation helps. It can help you respond appropriately. If you recall from Chapter 1, Kevin was wracked with jealousy, anger, and doubt during his wife's Internet chats with other men. His meditation was fragmented by painful emotions and memories. But he was able to use meditation to stop runaway thoughts—thoughts that kept him feeling that his world was falling apart.

As his breath calmed his mind, he could see that his wife had set boundaries she wouldn't let other men cross. He could see that she chatted on-line without an emotional involvement. "I was able to examine my insecurities in a detached, concentrated manner," he says. "I was taking something little and blowing it up." Until he focused, he couldn't see the reality. He could only see what his mind was making of it.

Kevin hasn't mastered mindfulness. But he has started down the path to using it to his advantage. As you sit and become more skilled, you can use meditation in the same way. You will get closer to seeing sensations, thoughts, perceptions, and emotions emerge. You will also get better at seeing your reactions. You may even catch them before judging, before grasping, before fearing, before acting. As you do, you will begin to make truly conscious decisions.

When challenged by the outburst of a student, one teacher says that meditation helped him handle his reaction. "I am aware ever so briefly of seeking out the quiet place in my mind whose availability I know from my daily sittings," he says. Even in that split second, "I. . . step back from the emotional charge and observe it or find a centered place. . . .I am able to respond in a more measured, thoughtful way, rather than an instinctive, reflexive way."

Your Prognosis Report

How fast can you expect such changes from daily sitting? Realize that you have probably spent decades piling on layers of reactionary thinking. You need time to shed them, and the build-up of stress they've caused. You should think of the process as you would peeling an onion. You have to proceed one thin layer at a time. And even as you shed the first, you may see little change. You may even feel worse off. This happens to some people as they feel hints of relief, only to grasp how many layers remain. You may feel discouraged. You may even feel stuck.

Rest assured that you're probably not stuck. Studies have shown that in as little as a few weeks you make some progress. Maybe a lot. In one study, about one hundred elementary, middle, and high-school teachers were asked to meditate for five weeks. They reported significantly lower perceptions of stress, anxiety, and burnout when they meditated only two to five times per week for twenty minutes.

Many people in the United States have entered formal mindfulness meditation programs. Along with the center run by Herbert Benson in Boston, one of the most renowned programs was developed at the University of Massachusetts Medical Center and is now taught at hospitals around the country. It was developed by Jon Kabat-Zinn. In this eight-week program, people with severe health problems learn to sit, walk, and move in meditation. On top of classes, each person is asked to practice forty-five minutes a day. This is a lot of meditating, but the results show the time invested pays off.

In a study in Connecticut, nurse practitioner Beth Roth interviewed patients who went through a mindfulness-based stress-reduction program. They had each attended her classes at the Community Health Center of Meriden. She asked about the program's benefits. Patients often said they were surprised how much they had changed in just a couple of months. They cited greater peace of mind, more patience, less anger, fewer temper outbursts, and better relations with family members. They also cited more restful sleep, greater self-knowledge, a greater sense of well-being, and more acceptance of aspects of life over which they have no control.

Everyday Meditation

Anchoring Breath.   Before reading further, meditate for the next minute. If you start thinking about what you've just read, note your thoughts and return to your breath. If you become aware of feelings or images, note them, too. Feel how, as your mind drifts, you can regain focus by pulling on the sensations of your breath. It's as if your breath is an anchor. Pull on it to come back to the center.

We can't stress enough how essential formal sitting is in your meditation practice. The quiet sit, for one minute or twenty, gives you time to build your skills with the fewest distractions. It is in a quiet, secluded sit where you can best grasp and solidify a sense of your breath as an anchor.

But remember that you can find the anchor of your breath in a lot of places far from your cozy corner at home. Fact is, you can find it anywhere, anytime. You can sit seven days a week, during any of the twenty-four hours in a day. The practice is available 24 x 7 x 52.

You may have trouble finding a convenient time to sit. We assure you that you'll have trouble if you simply try to hit the brakes in the middle of whatever you're doing. But we suggest you find natural pauses in your day. Pauses after innumerable to-do items. Pauses after phone calls. Pauses during bathroom breaks, coffee breaks, and lunch breaks. Pauses in waiting rooms, on buses, on planes, on trains. You don't have to stop the action to find time to sit. You just have to sit when the action stops.

Stay open to the possibilities. Craig Moser does. Remember he is the clerk to a federal judge. Craig sits for at least fifteen minutes each morning at home. But at work, if he feels his concentration waning, or feels nervous or overwhelmed, he meditates in his chair. His sit lasts for less than a minute. He may just count his breaths one through ten. Still, "It resets my bearings," he says. "It's a mental reset button."

Craig gets more daring at times. When court is in session, he takes a seat in front of the judge, facing the gallery. If the action stops, as when a lawyer and client confer, Craig can't go anywhere. He can't even turn around. So he meditates. He can't close his eyes, but he stares blankly at his papers and follows his breath. When he tires from a case with many pieces of evidence, he says, the quick sit refreshes him.

Kevin, as operations manager of a local utility, also takes time-outs for a sit. "If I can sit at my desk and control my breathing for even five minutes," he says, "it really helps clear my mind." But often he finds his employees interrupt him. Even when he closes the door, they knock. So he sneaks off to the restroom once or twice a week. In the privacy of the stall, he meditates for up to ten minutes.

You, too, can seize workaday pauses for one-minute meditations. How many times a day do you wait at red lights? In line waiting for a cashier? At the copy machine waiting for copies? At the front door waiting for the family? If you're stuck waiting, stop: Pull on the anchor of your breath. At many of these times, you can find a perfect moment to "sit" on your feet.

Of course, you'll have to adjust your technique. You can't sit in your car at a red light with your eyes closed. You can't wait in line without shuffling your feet. But you can narrow the focus of your attention to the rise and fall of your belly. You can mindfully ride the flow of breath in and out, in and out.

The irony is that ordinarily you may hate cooling your heels. Waiting may cause you inordinate stress. It may make you feel a bit like a penned hound—all you do is hanker to get on with the fox chase of life. Your mind, unoccupied with forward motion, paces back and forth. The "wait time" feels like "waste time." But remember: That's the menace of your one-minute mind. You can easily turn wait time into a one-minute meditation.

Troubleshooting

All of this can sound easy. The steps are so simple! But the steps hide plenty of challenges.

Sticky Thoughts

Giving undivided attention to your breathing sounds like a reasonable request. But you will soon learn that your mind divides your attention in more ways than you ever thought possible. What's more, it often channels your attention against your will. You may feel impotent in trying to meditate. You may think you're getting nowhere.

But hold on! It's normal for torrents of thought to blast aside your efforts to just "be." Take this as a signal to fine tune your sitting practice. If you have trouble focusing, try counting 1, 2, 3 on each in-breath and 1, 2, 3, 4, 5 on each out-breath. Taking longer out-breaths has a calming effect.

Remember, your attitude counts as much as your technique. Keep telling yourself: What comes up is O.K. The mind loves to chase new cars. Let them come, let them go. Just make an effort to be mindful. All thoughts exhaust themselves when the light of awareness shines on them.

Sticky Feelings

Along with persistent thoughts, you may encounter sticky emotions: desire, anger, sadness, restlessness, boredom, fear, doubt, drowsiness. If these feelings won't dissipate, try to observe them rather than letting them go. Shift your focus from your breathing to the feeling. Locate where the feeling resides in your muscles or gut. Where is the tension? The burning? The ache?

If you feel angry, say silently to yourself, "anger, anger." Then feel the clench of your jaw, the firing of the fine fibers in your vocal chords, the aura of heat in your mind. Focus deeply to find the source of the anger. Be totally aware of the riled bull surging into your head. Where does it come from? In the gentle light of mindfulness, the bull often lies down and rests. It doesn't spread the dust of reactionary thoughts across your consciousness.

Is focusing on an unpleasant feeling risky? Could the focus make it worse, endow it with more power? Actually, no. What gives a feeling power is pushing it away. Boredom, fear, doubt, anger, desire—if you try to banish them, your resistance empowers them and they return to hassle and haunt you. By focusing on their emergence, growth, and trajectory, you see that it is your mind that gives feelings power.

As Kevin Nuñez says, when he sits, he can look at anger more as a third party. He can judge better whether the anger is appropriate. He can see better ways to respond. "I have a real long fuse, but when I come to the end of the fuse, I really blow up," he says. With meditation, "It's like resetting the fuse." He reconnects to the anchor of his breathing and restores calm. "If I stay mindful, I can keep from losing my temper." Such an approach deepens your skill in quelling stress.

Itches, Etc.

As you're trying to sit, unmoving, you're going to feel an itch on your face. Or maybe a dull ache in your neck or lower back. What do you do? Resist the temptation to scratch or change your position. First feel the itch or ache. Like thoughts and feelings, itches and aches offer a chance to practice awareness. Note both your sensations and the reactions of the one-minute mind.

Be sure to feel the itch fully. Note how it pricks or crawls or buzzes or tickles. Feel it move. Note your impulse to scratch. Note your impatience for relief. Now when you can't stand it anymore, scratch! But scratch mindfully! Feel the movement of your arm with the attention you've given your breathing. Or if you ache, shift mindfully. Mindfulness of motion deepens your practice.

Your suffering, as meditation teacher Shinzen Young points out, is akin to the product of *pain* and *resistance*. He offers the equation: $S = P \times R$. What he's saying is that both the itch and your reaction cause consternation. Which causes more? When you can answer that question, you've become more mindful. (You may conclude, as Young says, that the equation should be $S = P \times R^2$. The resistance to pain causes more suffering than the physical pain.)

Goal Keeping

You can't help but have goals for your meditation. By now you probably have all kinds. Unfortunately, they encourage your mind to judge your efforts as a success or failure. The judging sets you up for creating stress, not getting rid of it.

The paradox of meditation is this: You are starting on a long-term program, but your focus must stay on the short term. You must focus with enough energy to work up a mental sweat—while not thirsting for a drink at the end.

This sense of nonstriving collides head-on with all that we've been taught. We normally set expectations for the future. We tell ourselves we're going somewhere. And we nurture the attitude that our reward is always ahead. But this approach creates a state of expectancy in meditation. And expectancy creates anxiety because you might curse yourself if you progress slowly.

Try to cultivate another attitude instead. When you sit, remind yourself that you've already arrived. Peace is within you. Peace is simply the mind's state prior to thinking. You're just setting yourself up to experience it more clearly. One way to view the experience of meditation is like the experience of a marriage or partnership. You don't go through life with goals of how deep or rich the relationship will become. You simply invest in the relationship because you believe in the partnership in the present. The depth emerges naturally, over time.

Excuses

Still, meditation demands some discipline. You can't read your way to peace. Nor can you talk or think your way there. You have to sit. And you can expect a daily struggle with procrastination. If you plan to sit for, say, twenty minutes each morning, you can expect a fight many mornings to get out of bed. When your mind feels fatigue, you can expect it to play all kinds of tricks to get you to skip your sitting.

But the alternative to summoning discipline is to let your practice lapse. There lies the danger: The longer the lapse, the less you feel you have invested. The less you feel you have invested, the less motivation you have to start again. In just a few days, you can lose your daily routine. And then the benefits slip away.

As one meditator says, "It's a real struggle for me to get out of bed. I can find a million excuses every morning." But the long-term benefits keep him going: "The chaos of the world still goes on, but it's much more manageable and in focus. I don't seem to be as upset or as worried about things. Meditation helps me in dealing with everyday or big life-time problems. I'm way more in the moment."

These rewards are open to all of us. They come to those who embark on a journey to master the one-minute mind. On that journey, we learn about the wily thought machine in our head. We learn about our hapless attempts to control it. We learn about our drive for clarity and harmony. We learn the skill for making that clarity a part of our lives. Our reward is that we empower ourselves to connect directly to the peace within us. Our only question becomes: Why didn't we learn this sooner?

Many skills for better living get little attention in our society. They rank behind many more tangible abilities—surfing the Web, writing a resume, pitching a baseball, barbecuing ribs. But we all deserve to learn at a younger age the techniques to cut stress and promote well-being. These skills belong on the educational roster of modern life. Everyone takes for granted learning the three R's to gain intellectual literacy. The time has come to learn early about using the breath to promote emotional literacy.

Meditative skills are not an adjunct to life. They're part of living skillfully. Focusing, concentrating, retaining presence of mind—these are valued by everybody. They serve all people, and for all time. As Paul Neary, the retiree we met at the start of the chapter, says, "I learned meditation in part because as long as I can think, I can still meditate. I can't change anything else, but I can still work with my mind."

Pen and Paper

New Day Resolution.   Mark a sheet of paper once again with the hours of an appointment calendar. Pencil in your meditation schedule for tomorrow. If you can, reserve at least one ten-minute spot for your basic sitting practice. Then mark two to three likely pauses during your day when you could insert a one-minute meditation. Now visualize carrying through on your appointments. You want to strengthen your resolve to take concrete steps to tap the drive for peace.

5

One-Minute Medicine

Healing is fundamentally mysterious,
yet open to conscious intention.

—ELLIOTT S. DACHER, MD

> **Warming Up.** Rest your hands in your lap, one hand over the other. Take three long breaths. Now while you follow your breath, focus on your hands. Imagine a beam of sun pouring onto them. Feel them heating. Feel the blood vessels relaxing. Invest all your attention in the sensation of your hands relaxing and warming. Do this for several minutes.

Did you realize you can warm your hands by simply willing it? Well, you can. You can coax your blood vessels to open. If you like, prove this to yourself by taping a thermometer to the fingerprint of one finger. In five to ten minutes of focusing on the notion of warming, you can probably raise your skin temperature by five to ten degrees. This is not magic. This is a proven fact from the scientific field of biofeedback. Most people can do it.

When you sit and focus on your breath during meditation, you do much the same thing. Why is this so? Because you're triggering the relaxation response. Your blood vessels relax and open. Arterial resistance goes down and the blood flow goes up. Vernon Barnes of the Medical College of Georgia actually measured how much. In a study on eighteen meditators, peripheral blood-vessel resistance fell 6.5 percent during meditation.

By trying to warm your hands, you're learning first-hand a key fact: When you sit, you exercise some control over the same systems you lose control over when stress gets the better of you—your nervous system, hormonal system, and muscular system. That these systems don't run entirely on autopilot may come as a big surprise to you. You can influence all three by using meditation. For centuries, many people suspected you could do so. Today, we know from medical research that it's possible.

What this means is that you can use meditation for more than calming. You can tap it to aid in healing. In this chapter, we will highlight a few of the more than one thousand scientific studies on meditation. Together, they offer evidence of how meditation can play a key role in restoring your health. They show that men, women, and even children who sit regularly can relieve a variety of disorders, ranging from heart disease to chronic pain to anxiety.

This chapter won't review all the studies of meditation. It simply paints a picture of the most reliable and common of meditation's benefits. We caution that no medical procedure, medication, or therapy works for everyone. Gathering enough data to *prove* anything in medicine is a monumental task. That's why only one in nine medical procedures has been proven through systematic research to be effective. But in the past decades, the studies of meditation offer convincing evidence that a sitting practice can alleviate many stress-caused illnesses.

This book isn't meant to encourage you to delay in getting a doctor's advice if you suffer from an obvious illness. If you're sick or feel unwell emotionally make an appointment with your doctor. Get enough facts to understand what ails you. Only after you've sought appropriate counsel from your doctor should you decide what role meditation should play in your treatment.

Remember one of the most appealing facts about meditation: In almost all cases it causes no side effects. If you usually turn first to medication to ease your ills, take the pluses and minuses of drugs into account. Many medications for high blood pressure, anxiety, and depression, for example, can cause impotence. If you have trouble with side effects, taking time to sit may work better than taking a pill.

One Teen's Stress

Our story about the healing powers of meditation begins with Candy Noonan. Candy is an eighteen-year-old high schooler. She faces typical high-school pressures. She strains to make good grades. She worries about writing research papers and essays. She struggles with math and science. She wants to be a doctor but needs a B average to win a scholarship. To her distress, she started 11th grade with a C average.

But Candy bears other pressures. She likes helping out when people ask, and has a hard time saying no. So she works in five clubs, among them the student council, her yearbook staff, and band. She has held the jobs of president, treasurer, and secretary. In the past, whenever others let work slip, she jumped in. "If I was the secretary, I was doing the president's job," she says.

Odds are that the stress of school and her habit of never saying no helped raise Candy's blood pressure. When she was sixteen, it hit 133/65. This is over the 95th percentile for her age, gender, and weight. Her weight also contributed to her raised blood pressure. At 5 feet 10 inches, she weighed 250 pounds. Making matters worse, she had what she calls "an attitude problem." She grated at the slights of rude classmates. And she has held that anger in. She took acetaminophen pills for headaches.

But Candy started meditation at sixteen. She began to meditate each morning and before tests. After eight months, she lowered her blood pressure to a healthy 105/58, which is normal. "Meditating helps you overcome things you were worried about," she says. She no longer needs pills for her headaches. Her average grade climbed to 84.7.

Lowering Blood Pressure

Candy's story shows one of the most widely recognized benefits of meditation: reducing blood pressure. Over the last thirty years, study after study has shown that meditation lowers blood pressure. This is big news. Why? Because people with low pressure live healthier, longer lives. A middle-aged man with normal blood pressure (120/80) is expected to live sixteen years longer than one with moderately high blood pressure (150/100).

An incredible one out of four adult Americans has high blood pressure. That's well over 50 million people. Many of these "hypertensives" run a huge risk. They can expect hardening of their arteries with fat deposits. With their arteries robbed of elasticity, they may suffer a heart attack, stroke, congestive heart failure, arterial aneurysm, or kidney disease.

A health problem of this scale is a national crisis. But, again, meditation can help, especially people with high readings. In the early 1970s, Harvard Medical School physician Herbert Benson was the first to show in rigorous experiments that meditation consistently lowers blood pressure. In meditators, Benson found that systolic (again, high-end) pressure fell from an average 146 to 137. Diastolic (low-end) pressure fell from 94 to 89.

A series of more recent studies (including the one Candy enrolled in) have since confirmed Benson's results. One study looked at one of the highest-risk groups, African Americans. Almost a third of African Americans suffer from high blood pressure. This study showed again that such hypertensives can reduce their blood pressure significantly. With meditation, the women's systolic blood pressure fell ten points. The men's fell thirteen. The women's diastolic fell six points, the men's eight.

Another major study that showed how well meditation works looked at people jogging on a treadmill. "Ambulatory" pressure, taken on a treadmill, foretells heart problems far better than the measurement of resting blood pressure. Scientists found that people who meditated had lowered their ambulatory diastolic pressure by nine points. Taken together, the results of these years of studies have been so consistent that in recent years one health-care organization after another has endorsed meditation for people with high blood pressure.

This news comes as researchers have reported another main fact: Meditation is associated with reduced atherosclerosis, the buildup of fatty material inside the blood vessels. The researchers looked at ultrasound pictures of the arteries of sixty African Americans with high blood pressure. After six to nine months of meditating twice daily for twenty minutes, the layer lining the subjects' carotid artery (the chief artery that passes through the neck up to the head) thinned by the same amount as for people taking lipid-lowering drugs (lipids include fats). Separate studies suggest that this amount of thinning has a marked effect: It drops the risk of heart attack by 11 percent and stroke by 8 percent or more.

If you've already had a heart attack or stroke, a sitting practice also helps. Consider Arthur Zell, age fifty-seven. Until recently, Arthur was a banker in rural Oregon. He drove three hours to work each Monday. He lived in a motel during the week and drove home on Thursday. He raised his kids "by telephone," he says. At work, he endured normal office stresses. He worried about loan losses. He would sometimes clash with his brother-in-law, the boss.

Four years ago, Arthur had a stroke (a sub-arachnoid hemorrhage). Arthur doesn't believe it was caused by stress. But he feels stress set him up for it. It wasn't just the stress of work. The main point is that he let stress get to him. "That stress of rushing and the frustration of driving—it wasn't always the big things," he says.

He had the stroke at his office. He was rushed to the hospital. After an MRI, doctors kept him in bed for nine days, four in intensive care. Fortunately, the hemorrhage healed itself. It damaged his brain cells only a little. Still, Arthur has discomfort in his head one or two times a week. He gets it from stress. And he gets it from, say, stooping to pick up sticks. At first, he says, "These little discomforts in my head were frightening."

Arthur found that meditation relieved the pressure. Now he sits each day. If he feels pressure, he stops and sits. "Twenty minutes works wonders," he says.

Quelling Severe Pain

Meditation can also help people with chronic pain. If you suffer such pain, you already know that doctors have no simple cures. Many things that work for one person don't work for others. That's in part because pain has, so to speak, at least two sides. One is the physical side. The other is the side coming from your mind. The physical pain itself hurts enough. But the mental anguish can hurt more. Chronic pain patients go through double agony in dealing with both.

The most research on meditation and pain has come from the University of Massachusetts Medical School. In 1987, a group led by Jon Kabat-Zinn reported on four years of work. Pain patients took Kabat-Zinn's eight-week meditation and stress-reduction course. They meditated forty-five minutes each day on their own. They also practiced doing yoga mindfully. (After the course ended, Kabat-Zinn found most people cut back on how much they meditate. Many sat just three times per week for fifteen minutes or less.)

Doctors use many scales to rate people's pain and mental anguish—a pain index system, an inventory of medical problems, an index of anxiety, and so on. Each system is standardized. Kabat-Zinn used these systems. He also asked patients to rate their own progress. Of 225 patients, one third said their pain was greatly improved. Another third said it was moderately improved.

At follow-up four years later, the patients' "present-moment" pain came back. That is, they said the physical hurt was no better. But their way of coping with the pain was a lot better. That is, by the standard gauges in one subgroup, more than a third of patients reported roughly two thirds drops in three symptoms: anxiety, depression, and hostility. People had apparently learned ways to relieve their mental anguish. They suffered less from the wailing of the one-minute mind.

Several studies show that meditation also helps with two specific but very different problems: psoriasis and pre-menstrual syndrome.

Psoriasis

Stress often triggers the onset or worsening of psoriasis. Many people think this skin ailment stems from poor skin growth. But just the opposite is true. The skin grows way too fast. It erupts with scaly, silvery patches or lesions. These often start on the scalp and worsen in winter. A common therapy for severe patients is standing naked in an ultraviolet-B light chamber. The light helps heal the lesions.

The isolation of the chamber makes a perfect place to test the value of meditation. A team again led by Kabat-Zinn did just that. They taught half a group of patients to meditate. They then asked them to meditate during each light treatment, guided by a tape. Nurses noted when lesions started to shrink, recede to half their starting size, and clear. The results: nineteen subjects cleared fully. Four did not.

Adjusting for fourteen dropouts, the team calculated that meditators had a 50-percent probability of clearing thirty or more days faster than nonmeditators. In one subgroup, that meant clearing in 83 days rather than 113. The results suggest that meditation can markedly speed skin-clearing for psoriasis sufferers.

Premenstrual Syndrome

Another health problem that doctors find hard to treat is premenstrual syndrome. PMS stems from many factors, such as diet and hormone imbalance. But cramping, irritability, water retention, and other symptoms worsen with stress. That made one medical team wonder: Would PMS respond to meditation? To find out, the team studied three groups of women. One learned to meditate. The second learned to chart PMS symptoms. The third was asked to read twice a day to relax.

After five months, those with severe PMS improved an average 58 percent with meditation. They had fewer emotional symptoms (impulsivity, low mood, anxiety, depression, social function). They had fewer physical symptoms (fatigue, water retention, cramps). And they rated themselves as better (more energy, less discomfort, better mood, and eating habits). The reading group got only 27 percent better, the charting group, 17 percent.

Handling Other Ailments

Meditation can probably alleviate other ailments. The most obvious are those caused by stress. Researchers and doctors have reported that sitting helps people with insomnia, asthma, infertility, high cholesterol, and headaches. Some reports show that meditators can slow the decline in a hormone linked with youth (DHEAS, a precursor of estrogen, progesterone, and testosterone). Further research will have to clarify, confirm, or replicate the results of these earlier studies.

Easing Cancer Stress

No research shows that meditation cures cancer. But studies do suggest that calming can aid in tumor fighting. Recall from the first chapter that stress depresses the immune system. It thins the ranks of the natural-killer cells that attack cancer cells. This suggests that a means to reduce stress could help cancer patients fight their disease. But this remains a hypothesis. One unpublished study shows that meditation can enhance the activity of the immune system.

We do know that meditation can help people stay mentally fit to fight disease. Cancer victims struggle daily with a range of emotional challenges. They worry about isolation from friends. They fret about contagion. They fear relapse, disability, job loss, and, of course, death. For these patients, any help to bear up under the mental burdens are a godsend. Meditation can help.

Gregory Montague, a Toronto lawyer, was told five years ago that he had non-Hodgkin's lymphoma, a form of cancer that infects the lymph nodes. But Gregory kept working. Meanwhile, he scoured the Internet and self-help books to learn how other people had beat their cancer. He also looked for alternative treatments.

About six months after his diagnosis, Gregory started a pill treatment. It didn't work. He still had swollen lymph nodes, fever, and anemia. It was then that he realized, "I need to do something to change my life and help me heal."

One thing he knew he had to change in his life was his stress level. In his job serving the elderly, he often faced crises. His clients were on the brink of losing pensions, housing, or health care. "It's a stressful job because you're dealing with people in stressful situations," he says. "You have to be a stone wall not to feel that." On top of job stress he had the stress from his disease. "The most obvious problem was the feeling that things were out of control," he says. "Your life is being taken away from you."

Near the end of the first year after his diagnosis, Gregory decided to try meditating. He was encouraged by a trusted law-school friend. As luck would have it, he felt better during the first sit. "It gave me a comfort level that was rather novel," he says. "It felt very, very good. It was such a tremendous stress reliever."

The meditation didn't drive Gregory's cancer into remission. But meditation did give him the ability to hang tough in his daily life. He had the energy to leave no stone unturned as he worked with his doctor to find the best treatment for his disease. He now meditates twice a day. He begins with twenty minutes in the morning and ends with twenty minutes on the subway on his ride home. "I find now when I get home I'm relaxed," he says.

The Mind Connection

Smiling Kindly.   Many people who meditate recite short phrases as they breathe. Often a few words laced into the breath deepen your calm. For the next minute, try a favorite from meditation master Thich Nhat Hanh: "Breathing in I calm my body. Breathing out I smile." (Or shorten it to, "In, calming. Out, smile.") As you recite, let a half smile come to your face. Focus on that smile.

What do you find? Does the half smile evoke friendly feelings? Most people find a bit of good cheer linked to smiling. As the smile brightens, so does the mind. Your smile, like your breath, connects mind and body. You can actually feel how meditation might have healing power beyond the physical. It can extend its influence to your mental and emotional state. Research confirms this intuition. Indeed, meditation can alleviate disorders of the mind.

Many mental ills don't call for a trip to the doctor. Take mild anxiety as an example. Studies show anxiety drops quickly with meditation. In one study, medical and pre-medical students learned to meditate in an eight-week course. Researchers graphed their anxiety and depression levels. The results: both levels fell sharply. The students' overall level of mental stress fell roughly by half (gauged by the so-called General Severity Index, or GSI).

A study of college students found much the same results. Mental stress (GSI) dropped by two thirds. (The anxiety part of the gauge fell 60 percent, the depression, 59 percent.) The students said they felt more in control of their lives. Yet another study of students found the more they meditated, the more their anxiety fell. Those who had meditated daily for two years enjoyed lower stress levels than those who had done so for less. They also did much better than those who had meditated for less than a month.

Anxiety Disorders

At some point, your anxiety may hit an extreme. You may feel like you're struggling to calm down like never before. You may have an anxiety disorder. If you do, you're not alone. As many as one in every dozen people suffers a disabling anxiety disorder at some time in his or her life. Among the disorders: panic attacks, social phobia, obsessive-compulsive disorder, post-traumatic stress disorder, and generalized anxiety disorder.

In a panic attack, you feel extreme fear or discomfort. The panic comes in peaks. You may feel like you are dying, going crazy, or losing control. In social phobia, you unduly fear humiliation and embarrassment. You don't want to go to social events and come in contact with other people. In an obsessive-compulsive disorder, you feel trapped into repetitious, often routine, thoughts and behaviors. In post-traumatic stress disorder, you reexperience traumatic events and their related stress. In a generalized anxiety disorder, you feel excessive and persistent anxiety lasting longer than six months.

Meditation may be a big help with at least some of these disorders. In early research, a team led by Herbert Benson studied thirty-two patients with anxiety disorders. After eight weeks of meditating, two thirds were better. They felt less tension and nervousness, and they also had fewer, shorter, and less intense anxiety attacks.

A team led by Jon Kabat-Zinn also studied patients with anxiety disorders. After taking the standard eight-week meditation course, patients scored significantly better on several anxiety and depression scales. When patients signed up for the program, thirteen of the twenty-two in the study said they had panic attacks the week before. After three months, only three reported such recent attacks. Three years later, patients had not relapsed.

The Cloud of Depression

Meditating can also help when you're depressed. Many studies report that meditators show fewer symptoms of depression. They also report that meditators show fewer symptoms of anxiety, which is often part of depression.

A pilot study at the Veterans' Administration hospital in Topeka, Kansas, found that 40 percent of chronically depressed veterans got a lot better after meditation. These patients had not responded to either medications or psychotherapy. They meditated in a group for five to thirty minutes once a day. Their gauges for depression and hopelessness fell by a third or more in ten weeks.

Improvement stems not just from calming, but from healthier thinking. Recall the case of Josh Bellemore, the dieting guitar player from Chapter 2. Josh's meditation teacher put his finger on the fix many depressed people are in: Josh's mind was flying repeatedly along the same negative flight path. That's why the teacher said Josh was like a moth. He was banging again and again on the same light bulb of mental anguish. He could find no way out.

Josh sees the problem today. "It was a debilitating feeling," he says. "By talking [from a depressed perspective], I was validating it." In hindsight, he adds, "Not being mindful makes you a victim of your thoughts and emotions. You're enslaved by them. You remain a victim unless you have some technique to divest of such thinking. You need some way to retrack the mind." For Josh, the technique was meditation. It helped him get off the scorching track of his one-minute mind locked in depression.

The most effective ways that therapists help people with clinical depression is with antidepressants and psychotherapy. In these cases, meditation may act as an aid to therapy. It works to soften the anxiety. It also elicits insight into mental ruts that strengthen depressive thinking. Maybe this is why recent research shows that relapse rates in depressed patients dropped in half when they learned meditation after successful treatment with talk therapy.

Curtailing the Draw of Drugs

Dozens of studies gauge the power of meditation to turn people away from drugs, tobacco, and alcohol. Many of them, using Transcendental Meditation (see Chapter 6), show that when people start sitting, they cut back sharply or kick the habit of chemical use and dependency. It may be that they find the well-being of sitting replaces the "high" of drugs. It may be that sitting dampens their drug appetite. Or it may be that meditation helps them recover from factors that underlie addictive behavior. Such factors include low self-esteem and feelings that life is meaningless.

In any case, studies in the 1970s by Herbert Benson show the rate of success many drug-dependent people experience in meditating. Benson tracked a group of nearly 1,500 young adults. The number still using marijuana two years after starting to sit dropped from 78 percent to 12 percent. The number using narcotics (heroin, opium, morphine, cocaine) dropped from 17 percent to 1 percent. The number using hard liquor dropped from 60 percent to 25 percent. The number smoking cigarettes fell from 48 percent to 16 percent.

These and a wealth of recent studies suggest meditation can have a marked effect. But many of the studies have weaknesses. The main one is that the subjects may have cut back on drug use anyway. Only more research will yield the data to say for sure. In the meantime, we suggest you view meditation not as therapy for addiction. It is an aid. It fits squarely into drug rehabilitation programs, like Alcoholics Anonymous, which call for meditation and prayer as a part of treatment.

Feeling, Acting, Performing

Besides showing the healing power of meditation, a number of studies suggest it can enhance the way we think and act.

They offer evidence that sitting regularly can sharpen our minds, improve our personalities, and help with personal growth. A lot of this research goes beyond the scope of this book. But a sampling shows the benefits that may prove healthful.

One claim for meditation is that it produces a greater sense that we control our lives. If we feel that people, events, and things force our lives down a trail against our will, we feel anxiety, anger, and depression. But when we feel in control, we feel better. We like to sense that we are blazing the trail of our own lives ourselves. Meditation can help you feel this way.

In a study of boys in a camp for juvenile delinquents, an eight-week course featuring meditation caused a significant rise in the boys' "internal control." As in many cases with meditation, the good results vanished when the boys quit sitting. In a study of high-school sophomores, a team led by Herbert Benson found that those who meditated in the group felt more in control of their lives. This came from sitting for fifteen minutes, three times weekly, at the start of health class.

Another claim for meditation is that it improves self-esteem. Together, low self-esteem and a feeling of external locus of control are linked with anxiety, depression, and disruptive behavior in children. Benson's study showed that by learning to meditate, children learn to have the power and ability to control their mood themselves, and thus boost self-esteem.

Many researchers claim that meditation can also improve concentration, attention, memory, and mental performance. In a study of nearly sixty college students, half learned to meditate. They sat for ten minutes at the start and end of each study session. Their grade-point averages rose from 2.77 in the fall to 2.93 in the spring. The GPAs of nonmeditators fell from 2.64 to 2.48.

How much meditation will enhance your performance is open to question. A lot more research is needed to say. But a bigger question remains: Can sitting help you lead a more fulfilling life? Can it propel you to more peak performances, peak experiences, or religious peaks? Some research suggests yes. But these journeys to peaks of peace are hard to document scientifically. If they interest you, we suggest you read some of the texts listed at the end of the book.

Meditation in Medicine

Body Check.   Take three cleansing breaths. Now scan your body for any prominent sensations—touch, tension, aches, itches, warmth. Start with your face. Work down through your neck to your shoulders. Feel the sensations within your chest and gut. Work down each arm and leg. As you note each sensation, ask yourself, "Where does the tension or itch or warmth come from? Is it from my body? Or from my mind?"

As you scan your body, you probably sense that some sensations clearly come from your body. Some others come from your mind. And still others come from, well, you're not sure. As for the body, some muscle tension comes from maintaining your posture. Some gut pressure comes from digesting your lunch. Some skin pinching comes from the pressure of sitting.

As for the mind, some facial tension, like furrowing your brow, comes from worry or strain. Some tightening and loosening of vocal chords comes from your voice box shadowing your mental chatter. Some of your abdominal tension comes from tensing your belly to hold your figure.

With each sensation you might ask, "Is it the mind or body from which it originates?" This is the same question you could pose when you're ailing from any serious health problems. The answer? Who's to say? Say you have chest pain. Is it from a heart condition? From an anxiety disorder? From weekday stress at home or work? Not only may you have trouble telling, so may a health professional.

That brings us to expand on a point we mentioned earlier. In the same way that you should scan for the root cause of your ailment, you should scan the possibilities for treating it. That means you should involve a doctor when you're not sure what to do. For people with serious illnesses, we don't recommend meditation by itself. It may help as one of several treatments. You have to integrate it in a program of care for your mind and body.

What that means is you may have to see more than just your family doctor. Research by Optum® of Minneapolis, a health-care organization, suggests that getting the best results often requires the advice of three different experts: a nurse, a counselor, and a family physician. Optum's research comes from data collected from its nationwide health and well-being hotline. The ailments Optum has determined as needing such integrated care include abdominal pain, depression, headache, chest pain, substance abuse, anxiety, panic, asthma, smoking cessation and eating disorders.

If you have a severe physical or emotional problem, spend some time with your doctor, nurse, or counselor figuring out the treatments that are right for you. To understand how vital this is, consider Sam Christy and Louisa Keniston again. Recall that Sam is a sixty-seven-year-old retired technical illustrator. Recall that Louisa is a forty-three-year-old

Bahaman bakery owner. Both suffer from high blood pressure. Sam had a heart attack at age sixty-four.

How should each treat their high blood pressure? As it turns out, very differently. Sam hoped to control his with meditation. He even cut back on $150 of medicine a month to see if he could. But Sam couldn't lower his blood pressure as much as he wanted with either medication or meditation. He could, however, stabilize it in the normal 135/70 range by following an overall healthy heart program of medication, diet, exercise, and meditation.

For five years, Louisa tried a variety of medications to treat her high blood pressure, three of which didn't work. Worse, they made her feel uncomfortable and made her heart palpitate. Two others that she still takes worked only a bit. When she enrolled in a meditation study, though, she finally hit on a solution. Her pressure fell from 160/110 five years ago to 130/72 today. Louisa's twice-daily sit turned her life around. "Meditation is part of my 'medication,'" she says. "I can't go without it."

The obvious lesson here is that everyone is different. If you're ailing, ask your doctor how mind and body can work together. In the meantime, you can use meditation as preventive medicine. If you're under stress day in and day out, sitting can help prevent stress from affecting your health. You may not feel like you need it daily. But when a bad day hits, you'll wish you had stayed in practice. Meditation should be a tool used to develop your mental skills in good health and bad.

Meditation in Talk Therapy

You may wonder if you can combine meditation and talk therapy. The answer is yes. To begin with, the calming of meditation helps with a whole range of mental health problems. Second, insights that come through sitting help you comprehend your mind. A therapist listens to your story. He or she helps you to see the pattern of your thoughts. Meditation reveals your story to you directly. Either process helps you heal and grow.

But meditation and therapy are not the same. The therapist helps you substitute healthy thought patterns for unhealthy ones. In meditation you don't substitute anything. You simply observe. Your distance lets you examine your emotions without stirring up chaos. As you cease rushing to the scene to create an emergency, the energy of your one-minute mind peters out.

The best way to see how meditation and therapy might work together is with an example. For the sake of showing a complete case, we combined the facts of two actual patients into one individual. Al Nelson, thirty-six years old and married, is a physical therapist. Most days, he complained of feeling sad. Anxiety and worry woke him at 4 A.M. He lost interest in things he used to enjoy, like sailing, hiking, and racquetball. His only source of pleasure was a nightly raid on the freezer for ice cream. He fell asleep aided by a few glasses of red wine.

Al was barely able to make it through the workday. It was a tremendous effort to do so. But working with people in pain took his mind off his own worries. After work, he collapsed in despair. He worried he would lose his job or marriage. He feared he wouldn't be able to provide for his two young sons. His wife tried to help and reassure him, but she felt frustrated, was at a loss for what to do.

Al seemed to isolate himself more and talk less. When alone, he cried. He sometimes wished he could just fall asleep and never wake up. He said he had felt this way twice before in his life. The first time was for four months, during high school. The second was for six months, during the year after college graduation. He said his mother and her sister had struggled with depression several times in their lives. As he told his story, Al's posture was slumped. His face looked dejected, and his voice was low and quiet. He fit the profile of someone with recurring major depression.

On Al's first visit to the psychiatrist, he was asked to take a minute in silence with his eyes closed. Afterwards, Al said his mind was full of worries the whole minute. He fretted about his health, his family, his job. He began to cry. He was asked if perhaps the worrisome thoughts made him feel worse. He learned the importance of noticing the action of the one-minute mind. Al needed to track his thoughts more carefully, to see if his thoughts were true and valid.

He was guided in scanning and relaxing his muscles, and focusing on his breathing low in the belly. After a minute of breathing in silence, he was asked what had happened. Al's face softened as he said he felt calmer. He was encouraged to practice this one-minute meditation at least three or four times a day. In subsequent weeks, Al said the minutes felt like islands of refuge. The islands grew as Al practiced for three, five, or ten minutes at a time.

He was seen weekly for ten weeks. He was taught to identify automatic negative thoughts, and to introduce realistic ones. He was asked to write daily in a journal to track his progress. Because Al's depression was severe, he was prescribed an antidepressant and advised to take it for six months to a year, after which he could taper off.

Within a month of combination therapy, Al felt back to his old self. Six months later, he tapered off his medication. He continued to practice his one-minute meditation at work. He also sat for twenty minutes every evening as soon as he got home. The mix of antidepressant, sitting, and talk therapy worked just right for Al. And though he is no longer in treatment, he feels like his daily sitting is important in preventing a relapse.

If you suffer from a disorder of this severity, meditation can ease your pain. Quick relief comes just from the relaxation response. You can then use the meditation as a way to examine your thoughts, memories, and attitudes. You can see how they affect your behavior, create moods, and cause pain. When you use meditation along with therapy in this way, you can change self-destructive habits. You will also see yourself—more than drugs or the therapist—as the biggest player in helping you get better.

Plain Old Good Health

The stories and research in this chapter show how meditation is strong medicine. It helps us detect illness. And helps to heal it. But a question remains: Can it restore full health? Many medical treatments reduce symptoms of high blood pressure or psoriatic lesions or anxiety. But they may not cure your illness. Nor may they get you back to feeling or acting normally. Somehow or other, you remain less than healthy.

This is a hard question for many kinds of medicine. Recall from the last chapter the Meriden Community Health Center. Nurse practitioner Beth Roth once tracked every patient's physical symptoms. She noted them both before and after her eight-week mindfulness meditation program. But she soon found that an inventory of symptoms didn't capture the data to answer this vital question. The inventory was too narrow. It showed that people's physical and psychological symptoms decreased after the program. But the decrease in symptoms didn't say enough about the quality of their lives.

Roth was the first to gauge the success of meditation with SF36 (Short Form 36). Used across the United States, SF36 is a questionnaire that asks patients to rate how they feel and function. Roth confirmed that people who started meditating not only experienced a significant reduction in symptoms. They got better in a lot of other ways—in social, emotional, medical, vitality, energy, and other categories. This is early evidence that meditation can greatly improve the quality of your life and overall sense of well-being.

Your Care of Choice

Meditation is an extremely safe procedure. As we said at the start of the chapter, only rarely does it cause negative effects. Some meditators do struggle with bouts of anxiety, depression, or agitation. They may feel overwhelmed with emotions. Or they may feel upset as they unearth repressed memories. Generally this is all a part of learning to see the mind with awareness. Working through these periods brings the meditator farther along the path to peace.

If you question whether meditation is right for you, talk to your doctor. In some cases, you might uncover psychological problems, and these you might work out best with the help of a therapist. That's not to say your therapist will not suggest meditation or medication to speed up therapy. But he or she will choose to apply each of them selectively.

Meditation is not a good idea in some cases. Experts do not recommend it for many psychotic, obsessive-compulsive, dissociative, depressed, schizoid, autistic, or narcissistic individuals. They also do not recommend it (at least not without psychotherapy) for relationship or communication problems, career and work issues, phobias or trauma. The best thing is to get good advice from a therapist for emotional complaints, or from an internist for physical complaints. Both can help you create a program of care that's right for you.

As Sam Christy, the retired technical illustrator, says, when it comes to healthy living, meditation "is a piece of the puzzle." Put together, Sam's puzzle looks a lot like that of many heart patients. For medication, he takes a beta blocker, a calcium channel blocker, and a cholesterol-lowering drug. He eats five fruits and vegetables a day. He splurges with a three-egg omelet on Thursdays. For exercise, he runs mindfully on the treadmill at the local gym. And for meditation, he sits three times a week for thirty minutes.

If you think you have a serious disorder, talk to your doctor about your needs. Whether you have a heart problem or anxiety, you may need a two-, three-, or four-part program like Sam's. In the meantime, you can rarely hurt yourself by making time to sit. Just breathe!

Pen and Paper

Mending Through Mindfulness. Check the benefits you're seeking. . . and the strength of medical research that supports them.

Health Problem	Proof of Benefit from Meditation
☐ High blood pressure	****
☐ Chronic pain	***
☐ Psoriasis	**
☐ Premenstrual syndrome (low mood, low energy, water retention, cramps, overeating)	**
☐ Headache (tension and migraine)	**
☐ Anxiety ☐ Panic attacks ☐ Generalized anxiety disorder ☐ Post-traumatic stress disorder	***
☐ Depression	**
☐ Drug, alcohol, and nicotine abuse and dependency	**
☐ High cholesterol	**
☐ Insomnia	*
☐ Asthma	*
☐ Infertility	*
☐ Irritable bowel syndrome	*

**** = Strong clinical proof, including many randomized controlled studies showing significant improvement.

*** = Moderate clinical proof, including studies showing significant improvement.

** = Some clinical proof showing some improvement. Further research needed.

* = Many anecdotal reports from doctors and patients showing improvement. Further research needed.

6

Different Strokes

*Happiness is not doing what you like,
but liking what you do.*

—LEWIS CARROLL

> **Peace in Words.** Sit comfortably, close your eyes,
> and breathe deeply. Now instead of focusing on your
> breath, focus mentally on two sounds. On the in-
> breath, silently say, "ah." On the out-breath say,
> "omm." Immerse yourself in the feeling of these two
> syllables. Keep on for a minute. Enjoy your peaceful
> inner voice.

What you've just practiced is "mantra meditation." This
is an ancient practice, as old as breath meditation. The
"mantra," a word or phrase, replaces the breath as the main
object of focus. For some people, it works just as well as the
breathing technique. You probably felt right away the
soothing sensation of your inner voice. If so, you have discovered that, like breathing, words can focus your mind,
and calm your body.

We chose these words carefully. "Ah" and "omm" are the sounds of calm and well-being. "Ah" is the sound of a relaxed sigh. "Mmm" is the sound of contentment. We heave an "ah" when we slouch into an easy chair. We hum "mmm" when we're savoring a moment. Omm, it turns out, is a universal sound of harmony. It mimics the hum of a tuning fork. Just the opposite is the sound of "ssss." The hiss mimics the sound of static, and can make you feel anxious.

The reason for this one-minute meditation is not to teach you ancient sounds. It is to open your eyes. In finding what works best for you, you can stick with breath meditation. Or you can pick another variety. Meditation comes in many flavors. Choose one to fit your tastes, personality, temperament, home life, and job. In this chapter, we cover a number of kinds. Check them out. You may want to use several regularly.

All these meditation techniques lead down the same path—toward helping you to focus and stay aware. Many people divide meditation into two groups. The first nurtures concentration, the second, mindfulness. But in practice, one leads to the other, concentration to mindfulness, and mindfulness to concentration. Together, they help you to vanquish stress and find well-being. They are the healthy duo.

To make meditation work for you, remember that you first have to reaffirm your intention to meditate each time you start. If you don't resolve to cultivate concentration and mindfulness, you'll just cultivate ritual. Each time you start, dedicate yourself to the notion, "I will turn my attention, over and over, back to present, real, concrete actions or sensations." Then you will learn to go beyond your reactive, preoccupied one-minute mind. Then you can learn to feel calm, grounded, centered, present, and wise.

Mantra Meditation

There are many kinds of mantra meditation. Some are as ancient as the "omm" form. But in the West, the best known is called Transcendental Meditation (TM). This is the style used by Louisa Keniston, the bakery owner, and Candy Noonan, the high-schooler. It's also the form that was embraced by the Beatles in the 1970s. TM is a refined mantra meditation revived by Maharishi Mahesh Yogi. To learn TM, you take a seven-step course and receive a specially chosen mantra from a certified teacher. The practice is to sit twice a day for twenty minutes.

Patty Pimental tells a typical TM success story. Patty, now forty-seven, began TM in 1970, when she was in college. She felt the stresses of her era and age: learning to live on her own and handle the rigor of college schedules. She was trying to keep her grades up, and deal with male-female relations and intrigues. And she was navigating a social scene filled with drugs.

As she sought her place in the world, meditation seemed like a natural thing to try out. It was the second semester of her freshman year. "At that age, I didn't know what to expect. I just wanted *something*," she says, to relieve stress and provide meaning in her life.

But Patty loved the practice the first time. "I just slipped into it. It was so natural for me." Her grades rose from Cs and Ds to As and Bs. And she felt much more settled. In fact, she liked it so much, she became a TM instructor. When she was thirty-nine she earned her law degree. Now she runs a law practice and teaches TM on the side.

The TM organization has cataloged more than 500 studies on the benefits of TM. Some of these show that TM works better than other kinds of sitting meditation. But

TM is not the only kind of mantra meditation. If you want to use a mantra, you can start on your own. Choose a favorite word, or choose a poetic phrase, saying, or prayer (such as the Thich Nhat Hanh's phrase, ". . . breathing out I smile"). Then immerse your attention in your mental voice. Whenever you notice thoughts, feelings, or sensations, bring your attention back to your mantra.

Fixed-Gaze Meditation

Just as you can make a mantra the object of your focus, you can choose a visual object: a dot, flame, symbol, or artwork. To start meditating, establish an awareness of your breath in the background. Then open your eyes and fix your gaze on your object. As with breath meditation, note sounds, thoughts, and sensations. If your mind wanders, return to your visual object. If you get sleepy when you meditate in other ways, fixed-gaze meditation may work well for you. It helps keep you alert.

Many people choose a flame as the object of their fixed gaze. Flames naturally draw our attention and calm our minds. If you're at home, light a candle in a corner. If you happen to be camping, add a stick of wood to the fire as it is dying out for the night. Sit in the darkened amphitheater of nature. Feel the rhythm of your breath as an anchor. Watch the curl and lick of flames. Note the quieting of your one-minute mind.

Meditating on Images

You can also close your eyes and focus on an imaginary visual object. Or you can imagine and focus on a scene. This is called visualization. People who use visual objects summon from their memory an image they find pleasing. It may be a flower, a bubbling fountain, a quiet room, an autumn landscape, or a breeze-rippled pond. They then imagine the experience with all their senses.

How does this work? Say you choose a rose. After you center yourself with your breathing, run your mind's eye over leaves, thorns, and blossoms. Smell the scent. Feel the satiny petals. Or instead picture the rose growing. Imagine a sprout emerging from the soil, thrusting skyward, blooming.

When we met Dot Smerciak, in Chapter 1, we said that the stress of her early work as an intensive-care nurse was so high that she had chest pains. Her solution? Meditate every day at 11 A.M. for fifteen minutes. But in foregoing her coffee hour, she doesn't take up breath meditation. She does visualization. "Before I go, I'm churning, I'm all riled up, I'm in high gear," says Dot. But afterwards, she's ready to take on her job afresh. "My soul is washed clean. Every part of my being is totally different, totally relaxed."

Dot does her meditation in a special darkened room set aside by the hospital for this purpose. She first breathes deeply while reciting a mantra: "Breathe in peacefulness; breathe out tension." She then evokes a peaceful scene of a beach or a mountaintop. She may even visualize herself floating in a bubble over a landscape of rivers and lakes. For the first seven minutes, she often leads other hospital staff in a guided meditation. In the background, she plays calming, meditative music.

One of the other people who meditates at the hospital has devised a favorite image of her own. She bases it on a vacation she once took to Fort Lauderdale. It was her most relaxing vacation ever. So she first pictures herself in her Fort Lauderdale hotel. She then imagines walking to the shore. She sees the waves and water. She feels her feet touch the sand. She watches people walking. She enjoys the pleasure she gets from holding and reading a good book. (She no longer remembers which book, just the feeling.) As she imagines all these things, she rotates her mental focus from one part of the scene to the next. And she stays with those feelings. "It's very relaxing," she says. "It keeps me on an even keel throughout the day."

If you saw the staff meditate at this hospital, you would notice one big difference from the practice we've described so far. They lie on their backs. Lying down is actually a second traditional meditation posture. Some people have trouble staying awake when they lie down. But lying down works well for others. If you have trouble falling asleep at night, you might try it yourself at bedtime. Two other traditional postures are standing and slow walking, which brings us to the next section.

Moving Meditation

Minding Movement.   Sit comfortably as you would for sitting meditation. Settle your body and mind with a few deep breaths. Now roll your head in a circle to the left. Then roll it in a circle to the right. Go slowly. Feel the stretching of your neck muscles. Repeat several times. Pinpoint each sensation and track its movement. You may feel strain, aching, or even burning. Notice how each sensation changes in strength.

Meditating in a still, sitting posture should be the foundation of your practice. Sitting while you keep a strong intention to experience "just now!" avoids the distractions of movement. But you can regularly add moving meditation to your daily practice. Moving makes a nice break for stiff muscles. It also helps you develop mindfulness in daily life.

After a few neck rolls, notice something else. Hold your head in one position. Note your thoughts. You'll find that once again different positions evoke different emotions. Lilting to the side may suggest a sense of wonder. Pulling back may suggest revulsion. Hanging your head forward may invoke sadness. Tune into a couple of these moods. This is part of strengthening the muscle of mindfulness.

You can apply meditative focus to any movement. Recall from Chapter 3 that movement in sports may even coax you into a meditative state. But beware. Do not confuse mindfulness of movement with a mind full of thought *about* the movement. You can distinguish the two by asking a couple of questions: "Am I staying present with the flow?" Or, "Am I just forming an opinion about it?"

If you say to yourself, "This feels good, or this is easy, or my head is screwed on wrong," you're hearing the one-minute mind talking. If you just feel the sensation, you are being mindful. This is called "bare attention," and it is the greater clarifier.

Movement as a device to build mindfulness is an old tradition in Japan. You may have heard of the arts of archery, swordsmanship, and the tea ceremony. In archery, the goal is not to score points. In swordsmanship, it is not to conquer others. In the tea ceremony, it is not to quench thirst. Instead, the goal is to train the mind. As the long-time student of archery Eugen Herrigel says in the classic *Zen in the Art of Archery*, "The marksman aims at himself and may even succeed in hitting himself."

So it is with all movement meditation. We are aiming at penetrating the one-minute mind. The movement is a means, as breathing and mantras are, to propel ourselves into the quiet mind. For some people, too restless or angry or anxious or sad to sit, movement may be the best way to meditate. It may make a vibrant object of attention—a more skillful means to reach the target.

Walking Meditation

Most meditators know walking meditation as an alternative to sitting. In formal practice, people alternate sitting and walking. But walking meditation is not like normal walking. When you walk the dog, you often walk mindlessly. When you walk in meditation, you walk mindfully. Don't be surprised if you find this harder than breath concentration. As Thich Nhat Hanh says, "The real miracle is not to walk either on water or in thin air, but to walk on earth."

You can do walking meditation in many ways. One that works well is to synchronize your steps with breathing. Find a fifteen- to twenty-foot lane to walk in. The lane can cut across your bedroom, your yard, or anywhere you feel you're not going to be bothered or make a fool of yourself. Stand at one end of your lane and find a steady standing posture. Hold your hands in front, behind, or at your sides. On your first in-breath, lift your right heel and swing your foot forward. Place your foot back on the floor as you exhale. Do the same with your left foot.

You are walking slowly. Very slowly. Perhaps 15 feet a minute. As you walk, dissect the flow. Sense the relief of pressure on the heel as you lift. Feel the increase on the toes. Feel the unweighting in your skin and the swing of your foot. As you put your foot down, feel your heels touch. Feel the touch roll down the length of your foot.

Just as you've learned to watch your belly rising and falling, learn to watch your feet rising and falling. If you prefer, focus on your whole leg. But pay attention! If your mind drifts, bring it back to your footsteps. Remember that you walk an awful lot in your life, so learning to meditate as you walk is a great opportunity to strengthen mindfulness.

Another way to walk is to do so even slower. Try to feel every sensation fully. It may take two or more breaths to finish a step. A third way to walk is much faster. Take two or three steps for each breath. Focus on your body's overall movement in tandem with your breath. If you're a mountain climber, hiker, backpacker, or runner you may already practice this sort of focus, called rhythmic breathing.

Note how walking meditation runs counter to your conditioning. How often do you think of going walking without a destination? But that's what you're doing in meditation. You're not walking to get anywhere. You are there. You're just trying to realize it. Many people find that walks in nature, away from life's chores and commitments, are especially rewarding. As William Wordsworth wrote in his poem, "The Tables Turned":

One impulse from a vernal wood / May teach you more of man, / Of moral evil and of good, / Than all the sages can.

Yoga Meditation

One of the most popular forms of meditative movement is yoga. You may know yoga as a stretching exercise from India. And in fact most people try yoga as a way to relieve muscle tension. But yoga comes from the same tradition as meditation. Done mindfully, it leads down the same path. While it enhances flexibility, coordination, and muscle strength, it also strengthens our calm and awareness.

There are hundreds of yoga positions, or postures. To make them a part of meditation, simply take the intention to use the movements and sensations as your meditative object of focus. Stretch into each posture slowly. Note the feel of each fiber in your body. If you feel a strain, don't pull too hard. Carefully and slowly test your ability to turn, flex, and relax. Explore your limits—feel your limits—as a way in which to stay mindful.

As with any other meditation, go about yoga with the right attitude. If you're trying to accomplish something or go somewhere, you'll progress slowly. If you simply try to pin down where you are right now, you'll do better. Ask yourself: "What am I witnessing?" Don't form an answer in words. That would be the one-minute mind talking. Just pay attention to the anchor of your breath, and become aware of how your body feels in the moment. Observe the answers directly in your body.

Here are five postures you can try. Do them on a padded carpet or a mat. See if you can follow each muscular sensation. See if you can keep in touch with your breath. As with neck rolling, note how, as your body perspective changes, your mind does the same. Hold each posture for up to a minute, or long enough to feel you've dwelt in the posture mindfully. Relax into each position, and breathe.

Sky Touch

Stand with your feet a foot apart. Gently lift the top of your head towards the sky. Then lift and stretch your whole body

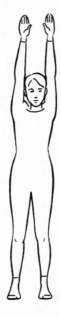

Sky Touch

upward. Now raise your arms slowly, as if you're letting them float. Point your fingertips to the sky. Hold for a minute, then slowly relax, letting your arms drift back down to your sides.

Hanging Loose

Now bend forward from the waist. Keeping your knees slightly bent, allow your arms, head, and torso to hang loosely toward the floor.

Shoulder Stand

Slowly bend your knees and squat. Hold for a minute. Now sit down and lie on your back. Pull your legs up toward your

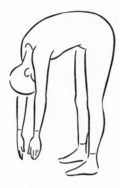

Hanging Loose

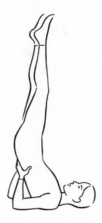

Shoulder Stand

chest and roll backward into a shoulder stand. Point your toes at the sky. Support your lower back with your hands.

The Plough

Let your legs fall over your head toward the floor. Hold wherever you are comfortable for a minute. Note the open-

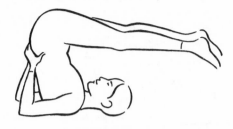

The Plough

ing in your neck and spine. Feel the lengthening of your hamstrings behind your thighs.

The Cobra

Return to lying flat on your back. Relax and roll onto your belly. With palms on the floor under your shoulders, slowly push up until your arms are almost straight. Arch your back and look at the sky. Hold for a minute. Then slowly return to lying flat. Breathe deeply and mindfully before getting up.

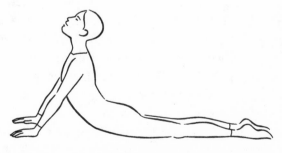

The Cobra

Meditate While You Exercise

Many people don't like the monotony of routine exercise. Biking, lap swimming, pumping iron, treadmill running, jogging—we all have a love/hate relationship with these daily regimens. We love the fitness; we hate the work and discipline. But with all of today's contraptions and exercise regimens, we have a great opportunity to double the return on our time. We can exercise and meditate at the same time.

If you want to try meditating while exercising, choose your sport with care. Some sports are so intense you have no chance to let your mind wander. You naturally stay present and aware. You might find that sports like tennis, basketball, or soccer work. But you may also feel too distracted with an opponent facing you. You may instead find that the solo, repetitive sports go well with the solo, sustained nature of meditation. You can more easily follow the rhythm of your breath, and of your limbs as they move.

If you exercise on a machine, you can probably even close your eyes as you work out. Start each session by, say, setting a watch alarm. Within a minute or so, you will be able to follow the inward gasp and outward heave of your breathing. If you lose track of your breath, try one of our favorite techniques: counting breaths to five, then to four, then to three, then two, then one, then starting all over again at five. Forty minutes of huffing and puffing three times a week will keep your heart fit. It can also keep your "good cholesterol" up. But the best part may well be the bonus time you enjoy for meditating and cultivating mindfulness and concentration.

Experiments show that meditation may actually help you breathe more easily and efficiently. Harvard Medical School's Herbert Benson asked people to ride an exercise bike while he measured their oxygen consumption. He adjusted their pace to keep a steady heart rate of 95 to 100 beats per minute. He found that when they began meditating they used 4-percent less oxygen. (Four of eight bikers used the same amount; four others used eight percent less.) We can guess that, as the subjects relaxed, they tended to use energy only in those muscles needed to do the work. They relaxed muscles tensed only from stress.

If you want to meditate while exercising, start by making a commitment to yourself to do so. Intention, again, is a springboard to success. Then fine-tune your practice in a way that works for you. Focus on your breath. Count your repetitions. Focus on sensations in your muscles. Observe and release your mental chatter. You will need some time to see what best helps you to concentrate.

Of course, aches, strains, joint clicks, and overheating can divert your attention. So can the side trips of the one-minute mind. You may feel you're not able to focus or stay mindful. But as with sitting meditation, practice counts for a lot. Eventually you will experience an odd and pleasant sensation: You will relax even as your muscles strain, even as you breathe heavily, even as you drip with sweat.

Meditating During the Day

As you've guessed by now, you can meditate while you do just about anything. That's not to say you should quit sitting. But you can approach all of life more mindfully. The next time you pop popcorn, eat one kernel like you'll never get another. Feel the initial crunch. Taste the salt. Feel the swallow. Stay with the kernel! In that kernel is the path to peace. In any daily activity is the path to peace.

The mundane tasks of life can become especially handy meditations. Brushing your teeth? Notice the feel of the brush, the taste of the toothpaste, the scrubbing movement of your hand. Start with the intention: "I will brush my teeth mindfully." (Who knows? Maybe you'll even feel like flossing!) Here are a few daily meditations from the people you've already met in the book:

Maria Borne (secretary): When Maria is working, she frequently reaches for the anchor of her breath. "I've learned to do it for a couple of seconds at a time," she says.

Craig Moser (law clerk): When Craig has to retrieve a file, he mindfully climbs and descends the stairs, much like mindful walking.

Kevin Nuñez (plant manager): When Kevin walks his dogs, he mindfully clambers over logs and stones on a beach along a nearby lake.

Arthur Zell (retired banker): When Arthur visits a public restroom, he mindfully dries his hands below the hand dryer (which usually runs for 45 seconds).

David Nichol (author): When asked to give a blessing before a meal, he leads a minute of silent meditation. And when hiking with friends, he encourages them to stop, listen, and feel their breath for a minute or two.

Sipping coffee, driving the car, washing dishes, doing laundry, taking a shower, you can choose to have the intention: "I will do this with 100 percent of my attention." Then just do it. A good idea is to choose one task to do mindfully each day—something you usually do on autopilot. This could be shaving, sweeping the floor, making the bed. Invest yourself fully in the task. Let nothing pass through the doors of your five senses without experiencing it. You'll find that chores you've considered a nuisance can turn into opportunities for better living.

The purpose of turning humdrum chores into meditation is to spread mindfulness into the mindless corners of your life. The more you live moment to moment, the more pleasing your absorption in life. The more pleasing your absorption, the less you feel stress and anxiety. Bad things don't bother you so much. Good things give you more pleasure. Imagine how much pleasure you miss in mindlessness each day? What do you miss when you wolf down lunch? Or when you gobble that popcorn?

Let's look at a more complex example of bringing mindfulness to daily living. Alison Lundberg, a twenty-seven-year-old real-estate agent, long resisted meditation. She recalls that when she was sixteen, she was in constant motion. She was so energetic that a good friend (a regular napper) bet her she couldn't sit still for ten to twenty minutes each day. She took up the challenge, though she felt it was stupid.

"There wasn't anything I could desire to do less than doing nothing," she says. "At first I was just determined. Whatever the challenge was, I could do it." But she lasted just a day and a half. "He was right. I just could not sit still," she says.

There is a little bit of Alison in all of us. Learning to sit still is not a goal that we naturally aspire to, or value. Time is too valuable to waste in idleness! But what we often don't see is that sitting still and sitting idly mean different things. In sitting still, we can build mindfulness. In sitting idly, we often fall prey to the willy-nilly travels of the one-minute mind.

Not surprisingly, the prime outlet in Alison's life was an active one: dance. She started when she was five years old. She had to work hard, though, and was always nervous in class. "I felt badly if I couldn't do something really well," she recalls. Dance did not come naturally. She set goals, and continually thought ahead about every move. By force of will, she became a competent dancer. She even went on to dance as a pro in New York, after she finished college.

For years it never occurred to Alison that dance could offer far more pleasure in the present moment. Partly what slowed this realization was that her teenage life was not a contented one. "I felt at that time very out of control," she says. "I was always wanting to be conscious every minute of the day. . . . I didn't want anyone to surprise me." She was so intent on controlling her mind and her life—rather than letting her parents do so—that she struggled with teenage anorexia nervosa, severely limiting her diet. "I wanted to be in ultimate control," and with anorexia she was, in a sadly roundabout way.

Alison's turning point came in an unexpected way. She had to stop dancing every day as she started a career in real estate. To make up for her days of lost dance, she started yoga. To her surprise, the course ended with meditation. To her greater surprise, she began to enjoy it. Those ten minutes of meditation became her favorite part of yoga. She began to see that control can come from some place other than wrestling the one-minute mind into submission. It can come from letting it go.

What Alison found—and it took twenty years of maturing to do so—was that meditation helped her let go of her obsession with control. Her yoga, meditation, and dance then grew together. "Today I feel like a whole different person dancing," says Alison. "It's the difference between moving with determination and moving with intention." Now she becomes so mindful she sometimes feels like she's getting lost in dance.

This is the power of bringing mindfulness to our daily lives. It works in two wonderful ways. It expands our joy while we sit formally. It deepens our pleasure in all the things we do in life. As Alison says, she's stopped thinking so much about the right and wrong way to dance. She's stopped setting so many goals. She has started observing the wonder of the action.

"I've been doing this same motion for seventeen years," she says. "I just started to appreciate how my toes feel, how my legs feel to stand on. There is a joy in dancing for me now that I never had before."

Spiritual Beginnings

In Spirit.   If spiritual or religious beliefs play a role in your life, choose a keyword that is especially meaningful. You could try *Jesus* if you're Christian. Or *Shalom* if you're Jewish. Or *Allah* if you're Muslim. Or *Sat Nam* if you're Hindu. Or *omm* if you're Buddhist. If you're not religious, choose a word like "one." Meditate for one minute with this word as a mantra. Repeat it over and over with each breath.

For most people, a spiritual mantra evokes a series of associations, images, feelings, and thoughts. It turns the mind not just toward calming and quieting and self-knowledge, but also to a receptivity to a greater power than ourselves. Do you get this feeling? If so, you are not looking just within yourself anymore. You're looking within and beyond and above. (To what, you may not be sure.)

One of the great stresses in life is the sense of separateness. As humans, we often ask questions like "Why am I here?" or "What is my purpose?" or "Who am I?" or "How am I connected?" We struggle with explaining and rectifying our sense of aloneness in the universe. If we feel disconnected, we feel anxious. If we feel lost, we get scared.

We naturally yearn for a link with a group—with loved ones, with family, with a community, with a nation. Nothing could be more human. If we're religious or spiritual, we seek to clarify and strengthen our link with others and with a higher power or being. Of course, not everyone experiences this yearning, but certainly many of us do. If you're in this camp, you'll wonder: "How does meditation fit in? Is it compatible?"

No matter what your beliefs, the practices in this book can enhance your spiritual life. To begin with, as you improve concentration, you clear away worldly clutter in the one-minute mind. The more enduring truths of existence stand out. For many people, these truths include a clearer sense of their God.

A scattered mind cannot be a spiritually engaged mind. A clarified mind opens a clearer channel to spiritual understanding.

Meditation in recent centuries has been associated more with Buddhism than other religions. And that is no doubt because meditation is a central practice in Buddhism. But the myth persists that the Buddha somehow invented meditation. (He just refined it.) Or in meditating you are somehow professing a new faith (probably to a cult). Not true! Especially as a beginner, you are merely learning a universal mental technique, which plays a role in nearly all religions.

Janet Fulgoni, a forty-five-year-old Web site designer, is Catholic. Janet began meditating after a series of tough, stressful events in her life. She suffered through a number of years of grief when her father died. She suffered from debilitating worry in her job as a bus driver after a drug-abusing passenger assaulted her. In turning to meditation,

Janet was not looking for a spiritual path. She was looking for a way to ease stress.

How does Janet link Catholicism and meditation? She is a devout Catholic, so this is a serious question. Before her Web business took so much time, she went to mass every day. "If I didn't have the Lord in my life, no matter how much I meditated it would be meaningless," she says. "I would never have any quality time without that half of the equation. If I felt I had to do meditation without religion, I wouldn't do it. I'm not pushing any thoughts of Jesus out of my mind."

But her approach is simple: "In meditation, if the thought of Jesus enters my mind naturally, I'll praise him," she says. "And then I'll go back to my breathing . . . When I praise the Lord, I feel blessings. So receiving a blessing from the Lord, and also feeling this relaxation and quiet [from meditation], is a bonus." Janet now meditates three to six times per week for fifteen to thirty minutes.

For some people, meditation plays a more active role in their spiritual life. In every major religion, monks, mystics, and saints have practiced meditation over the millennia to experience the truths of life directly. As the famous twenti- eth-century Catholic monk, Thomas Merton, said: "Meditation is for those who are not satisfied with a mere- ly objective and conceptual knowledge *about* life, *about* God—*about* ultimate realities. They want to enter into an intimate contact with truth itself, with God. They want to experience the deepest realities of life by *living* them."

What does living the deepest realities mean? That's a question for all of us to answer on our own. Meditation is a tool to improve the odds of our succeeding. Each major reli- gion hints at the same theme, though: You can aspire to real- izing a connection to something greater than yourself *on your own*. Out of the silence of the meditative mind, you can *feel* this union, a union with your God. This may be hard to put in words, but this sense of union can help resolve a deep—sometimes the deepest—source of angst in your life.

In this book, we don't tell you how to perform traditional Christian, Jewish, Muslim, or any other religious meditation. Each faith has its own meditation tradition better explained by others. But below we suggest some simple means to dovetail the kinds of meditation we have described with your faith. We think you'll find, like Janet Fulgoni did, that meditation deepens the spiritual feelings that may make up the most treasured part of your day.

For Christians

The desert fathers of Christendom, monks living in the deserts of Egypt as far back as the fourth century, developed a kind of mantra meditation still in use today. They recited over and over the Prayer of Jesus: "Lord Jesus Christ, Son of God, have mercy on me." You too can recite this prayer to deepen your concentration and sense of connection. You can also choose a biblical passage, such as scripture from the Psalms. If you're a Catholic, you may find more meaning in the Rosary if you recite it with the help of your meditative skills.

On a more modern note, you could take a cue from a Baptist meditator we know. A deacon in his church, he actually loaded a scriptural screen saver on his computer at work. He periodically sits back for three to five minutes to focus on the scripture's meaning. "Meditation really helps me develop a better line of communication with my Lord," he says.

Another means of using meditation is visualizing a scene from the Gospels. Put yourself in the scene. You are with

Jesus as he gives sight to the blind men. Make the scene come alive in all its emotion and power. As you view it in your mind's eye, you will deepen your sense of your relationship with God. The sense Christian meditators gain is not one of being alone. It is one of working to develop a shared sense of recognition and love with God.

For Jews

The approaches possible for Jews follow a similar pattern. Among the suggestions of Rabbi Aryeh Kaplan, who wrote extensively on meditation in the last century, are two. One is to recite the Amidah, the prayer recited three times daily, as a mantra. Since the first three sections are always the same, Kaplan urges Jews to memorize them (in Hebrew). He even notes that the first paragraph, only fory-two words, can be used alone as a mantra.

A second idea is to slowly repeat the Shema, the most ancient Jewish prayer, as a mantra. The Shema is only six words: *Shema Yisrael, Adonoy Elohenu, Adonoy Echad* (Listen, Israel, Adonoy, our God, Adonoy is One). You may recite the Shema slowly, taking seven to ten seconds per word, to make a one-minute meditation all on its own.

For Muslims

For Muslims, the approach can once again be similar. For relaxing and focusing, remember to center yourself with the rhythm of your breath. The most accessible way to dovetail meditation with Islam is to recite the *Shahadah*, the daily profession of faith, as a mantra: *La Ilaha ilia Allah, Muhammad rasul Allah!* ("There is no God but the One God, Allah, and his prophet is Mohammed.")

We don't suggest you replace your regular religious practice with mantras and breathing. But the ritual of religion, like much ritual in life, can lose its freshness and force when it becomes automatic and reflexive. With meditation, you can bring mindfulness into your spiritual practices. You can respond to the ancient words of your faith with newfound energy. You can understand them with new depth. Ultimately, your aim is to strengthen your connection to the larger-than-life power around and within you. This connection is made stronger with each moment of mindfulness.

What this all suggests is that meditation can, for everyone, lead far beyond stress relief. It leads to a place where we feel less isolated and adrift. Our sense of scatteredness transforms into a sense of being together. Our sense of aloneness transforms into a sense of oneness. We find meaning in our practice, and we find more meaning in everyday life.

Making our way along this path—whether spiritual or secular—is a stress reliever of the highest kind. But it is much more than that. It is an aid to transcending the one-minute mind. And by transcending—or in just making the effort to do so—we discover healthier and happier living.

Pen and Paper

Meditations for All Minds.   You may be a breathing "loyalist." That is, you may find that you enjoy and benefit from basic breathing meditation. If so, you're in good company. But you may also find that other kinds of meditation work well. Here's a guide to meditations for different moods. Put a check by all those that appeal to you. Try them when the time is right.

IF YOU'RE . . .	TRY . . .
☐ Mildly Stressed or Anxious	. . . sitting with your eyes closed counting breaths in a quiet room.
☐ Distraught	. . . sitting with a mantra: "May I be happy. May I be peaceful. May I be at ease." As you feel better: "I am happy. I am peaceful. I am at ease."
☐ Depressed	. . . brisk walking meditation outdoors, in a natural setting . . . or cleaning your house mindfully.
☐ Scattered	. . . five minutes of yoga stretching followed by breath sitting, counting out-breaths one to five.
☐ Angry	. . . vigorous exercise followed by 30 minutes of sitting.
☐ Unconfident	. . . imagining the scene that most worries you. Then using breathing meditation with a mantra: "I am strong. I am confident."
☐ Burned Out	. . . a short, brisk walk, and then 20 minutes of breathing meditation.
☐ Lonely	. . . meditating with a friend or group. Start your own meditation group at your home. Invite people to bring readings and snacks.
☐ Restless	. . . sitting while you scan your body for sensations, or fast walking mindfully.
☐ Seeking Meaning	. . . reading a few minutes from a spiritual book, before or after sitting.
☐ Fearful	. . . imagining a safe place and inviting teachers, mentors, and loved ones to sit with you there.
☐ Can't Sleep	. . . scanning body from feet to head and back down again, relaxing and softening the muscles along the way. If you can't sleep after 20 minutes, get out of bed and read until sleepy.
☐ Bored	. . . meditating on an image of your body in flow, and then acting out that image.
☐ Hungry	. . . breathing meditation with noting of sensations . . . or walking meditation . . . or preparing a meal and eating mindfully.
☐ Lustful	. . . sitting and mindfully observing any fantasy that unfolds . . . or making love mindfully.

7

The *New* One-Minute Mind

*Right now!. . . It is possible in this
moment! It is this moment!*

—SHUNRYU SUZUKI, ZEN MASTER

The phone call knocked Carl Crompton for a loop. A sales
and marketing manager for a Missouri electronics supply
firm, he was in New York City on business. His fiancée had
been on the line, and she had bad news. She'd taken off his
ring. She'd broken their engagement. She left him with
words that burned like acid into his torn heart: "You are
just so intense!" she said.

Carl, twenty-five, hit bottom. "I was walking in New
York City in a complete daze," he says. "I was really hurting." Hurting so much that, when he got back home, he
saw a social worker for emotional help. "I was tripping out
about this relationship."

That was when he learned to meditate. And he then
started to realize just what his fiancée had meant. He began
to see the dark side of his "success-oriented, hardworking,
hard-driving" thinking. What he found is what you've been
finding in this book. Meditation takes you on a journey. It
starts as you learn about the one-minute mind. It ends as
you develop skills to cultivate a *new* one-minute mind.

For Carl, the journey began as he started to see how his mind worked. He was plagued by worries that he had too much to do. He was anxious that he couldn't do what he wanted. He feared that he'd be a failure. He found, he says, "There's all this muck in my brain. It's overloaded, confused, fatalistic, panicky, torn," and has "lots of questions and not a lot of answers." His mind dwelled in the past and the future, and rarely settled into the present moment.

When he started, Carl meditated twice a day for a year. Paying attention to the workings of his mind calmed him. Observing the patterns of his thought put the drama of his life in perspective. "It's unbelievably powerful if you can watch the way the mind behaves," he says. "Having the ability to have an outsider's view of myself tends to temper me a lot."

Now, three years later, he feels he has new tools to stay relaxed and even-tempered. "My life is so much more at ease," he says. When he gets stressed about sales budgets or losing a sale, he takes a few deep breaths. When he pushes himself to the point of feeling burned out, he sits for twenty to thirty minutes. "I know there's this place I can go if I really need to," he says. "There's this goodness inside me. There's this special, peaceful spot I can find."

Mindful Thinking

The journey from the one-minute mind to the *new* one-minute mind is a journey from mind as victim to mind as victor over mental turmoil. As you embark on this journey, you will find, as Carl did, that pleasing changes take place. As you sit, as you relax into the moment, you feel better bit by bit. You act better. You think better.

When your mind doesn't splinter your attention into so many parts, you're able to experience life more as a flow. A little space creeps in around each thought. A little time passes between each of them. You don't feel as though one thought is always crowding out another. You feel like you have more room to respond mindfully. This is one of the early rewards of the new one-minute mind.

As you improve your meditation skills, you experience more moments unbroken by judgment. Unbroken by fear. In the past, you may have felt as though your thoughts tossed like foam on the surface of a wind-whipped lake. Your mind may have felt turbulent, murky. But with sitting, the surface chop quiets down. The murkiness settles. Your mind more often lets you experience each moment as it is—reflecting reality like the surface of a placid lake.

What you begin to gain is a clear mind. And with that mind, you more skillfully see into the depths of your self. You see the one-minute mind at work. You see your thoughts emerge. You feel your mind and body react. You observe your impulses to run away from the present moment. So you gain insight into how you experience living. How your life endures for so little time. How it changes so swiftly. How it challenges you day in and day out.

With insight, your mind becomes more accepting. Accepting of yourself. Accepting of each turn of events. Accepting of things you can't change. Accepting of friends and foes. An accepting mind feels that this moment, this circumstance, this person, this part of life is O.K. When your mind is accepting, you feel less discomfort from desire. You stiffen less with anger. You surprise yourself with humor.

The accepting, meditative mind deepens your sense of fulfillment, and of contentment. Feeling better on the inside, you can more often turn your attention to the outside. You give more freely to others your attention and understanding. You're more able to find the best in other people. And the best in each moment. More often you find that other people find the best in you. In an uncanny way, your way of behaving starts to swing events in your favor.

As you enjoy these subtle mental rewards, you also find what means most to you in your life. As the mind quiets and you observe the deep waters of your thought and emotions, you sense more acutely what makes you happy, what makes life satisfying. Accumulating possessions and experiences fades in importance. You find you can use meditation to access and reconnect with personal truths—the truths that help you shape your outer life to match your inner one.

Your New One-Minute Day

Take a moment to imagine a day in your life as a one-minute meditator. As you awake, you lie still. Into the stillness you let emerge your sense of the present moment. You note your breathing. You sense the delicious feel of the sheets. You note fading images of dreams. You watch thoughts emerge as the machinery of your mind clicks into gear. You enjoy all of this with a sense of ease.

After a few minutes, you begin your waking day on a chair or cushion for meditation. This is a special place. You might spend ten minutes here, or twenty or thirty if you can. Your intention to sit and your practice both set a tone of mindfulness for the day. You enjoy carrying that tone to the shower, to the breakfast table, to kissing loved one(s) goodbye, to driving or walking to work. As you commute, you make an extra effort to notice: breathing, sensations, sights, sounds.

The day flows more easily when you're mindful. As you remain calmer, feeling less conflicted, less doubtful, less self-critical, you free up energy to work more effectively—on your own and with others. You enjoy staying busy but you don't let busyness burn up your mental energy. When stress builds in the forehead, shoulders, or lower back, you take a minute to calm yourself. When you find yourself gobbling snacks, you pause to taste subtle flavors. When you catch yourself talking without end, you pause to listen and observe.

At the end of the day, at home, you return to your seat for a short sit and take a few minutes to shed stress from work. Your family or friends may hint at how sitting has made you more easygoing. Three times a week, you also exercise. At dinnertime, you mindfully chop vegetables, pour drinks, lay out the silverware. You speak to your family with awareness. You listen attentively. You notice colors, textures, and smells as you savor the unfolding evening. At bedtime, you end the day as you began—feeling the delicious sheets, relaxing your whole body, minding the rhythm of your breathing, floating your mind in stillness.

The one-minute meditator's day ends. It's a routine day, but it is not crowded with routine perceptions. It's a busy day, but it isn't filled with busyness of mind. It's a day in which you feel calmer. A day in which you find more meaning in every minute. The one-minute meditator's day is a day for which many of us yearn constantly.

Your One-Minute Roadmap

The journey to get to the new one-minute mind isn't easy, but the path is plain. You don't need to find a guru to start on the path yourself. You don't have to become a guru to help others start on the path, especially with a one-minute meditation. Let's look at the path again briefly.

- The One-Minute Mind. At first, we sit and see the avalanche of thought and emotion tumbling through our heads. We realize our enslavement to unhealthy, repetitious thought patterns. We see that we act, and react, out of habit. We realize we rarely live in the present moment. This habitual mind is a stressed and anxious mind.

- The One-Minute Escape. We also sit to see how we seek relief by chasing solutions outside ourselves. We spend endless time hankering after pleasure and skirting displeasure. We distract ourselves with TV and work. We stop stress with drink and drugs, and risk addiction—often putting ourselves in a downward emotional spiral.

- The Drive for Peace. As we look deep inside ourselves, we see that enduring relief lies within all of us. We've experienced places of peace already, indirectly—in sports, in nature, in our faith. We've revered these moments, moments of pure contentment. They all are the result of being absorbed in the present.

- One-Minute Meditation. We learn that we can experience more of these special moments *directly*. We can access them through meditation. With this simple mental technique for calming the mind—"sitting"—we can find equanimity in all that we do. We can momentarily free ourselves from the one-minute mind. Sitting lifts us to a place of awareness, stillness, and healing.

- One-Minute Medicine. We've examined the medical research that has shown we can tap meditation to aid in healing. As we sit to stop stress, we realize we can also restore the fitness of our minds and bodies. We can slow the hardening of the arteries while we soften our attitudes and still our minds.

- Different Strokes.   We've explored new kinds of meditation and have learned we can use them to enjoy the same relief as formal sitting. We've discovered, however, that we must hold the intention: "I will sustain moment-to-moment attention on the here and now!" At no time of the day do we need to go without the help of the calm and the insight we earn through meditation.

- The New One-Minute Mind.   Our journey shows us that we can take simple, concrete steps to move our minds in the direction of peace. No special skills are required. We can find a place of calm on our own. This is the place where we can just "be" with our minds and bodies in action throughout the whole day. Returning to our place of awareness of breathing helps us build a healthy sense of self.

Getting Started

From the stories of all the people in this book, we've learned how to travel the route to the new one-minute mind. And now is the time for you to travel that route by yourself. Along with all the meditators you've met in this book, take inspiration from Joan Lunden, the popular former co-host of ABC's morning news show, *Good Morning America*. Lunden tells how her busy life a decade ago ravaged her emotions. She tried to control everything—her job, schedule, marriage. But they all ended up controlling her. It was through diet, exercise, and meditation that she let go enough to ease her stress. What did she conclude? "A day isn't a good or bad one because of what happens around you," Lunden writes. "If you can stop reacting to events, they will no longer determine whether a day is good or bad—you will."

Take the time to use meditation to turn more bad days into good days. Sit to understand the one-minute nature of your mind. Sit to see how you think, minute by minute, in unhealthy ways. Sit to see how you escape, minute by minute, in repetitive, unhealthy distractions and diversions. Sit to see how you yearn, minute by minute, for a more lasting sense of peace. And after embarking on this journey, learn how you have the power to relax into, at any minute, a state of enduring contentment.

Don't let weeks, months, or years tick by without pursuing your place of contentment. Don't put off that satisfaction until after work. Don't let it go until the weekend. Don't put off contentment until you've retired. Resolve to find it today, in every minute. Do it for your mind. Do it for your body. Make it a part of healthy living. As your doctor might say—"Meditate 2x daily."

The new one-minute mind—this is the elusive goal of all of us. Yet it is a goal that is constantly accessible, and ultimately available. Begin to attain it by setting aside your first minute—just one of the 1,440 in a day. You now know the way to begin—just breathe! If you haven't started already, sit today, this minute. "Be like a lion," as meditation teacher Thich Nhat Hanh says, "going forward with slow, gentle, firm steps."

> A mindful minute is a well-lived minute.
> A mindful day is a well-lived day.
> A mindful life is a well-lived life.

Last Breath.   Sit comfortably, close your eyes, and just listen. Listen intently. Feel the sensation in your arms and legs, and the touch of your skin against your clothes. Note spots of tension, in your shoulders and face especially. Allow your muscles to soften. Now watch your breath with fresh awareness. If your mind is busy, count your breaths, one to ten. As your belly swells, as your nostrils fill with air, you return closer to your center, your place of peace. Linger there. Enjoy. After a minute, or ten or twenty, mindfully resume your day.

Pen and Paper

Clocking Your New Mind.   Take out your picture of a clock from Chapter 1. Look at all those gray slices. Those are the slices of mindless activity. Now choose two of them. Resolve to bring mindfulness to at least a portion of each slice. Highlight the new moments with a bright marker. You have begun to see the brighter face of your new one-minute mind.

Further Reading

Aitken, Robert. *Taking the Path of Zen*. New York: North Point Press, 1982.

Benson, Herbert, M.D. *The Relaxation Response*. New York: Avon paperback ed., 1990 (originally published by William Morrow, 1975).

Boorstein, Sylvia. *It's Easier Than You Think: The Buddhist Way to Happiness*. San Francisco: HarperSanFrancisco, 1995.

Borysenko, Joan. *Minding the Body, Mending the Mind*. New York: Bantam paperback ed., 1987 (originally published by Addison-Wesley).

Gallwey, W. Timothy. *The Inner Game of Tennis*. Revised ed. New York: Random House, 1997 (originally published in 1972).

Hanh, Thich Nhat. *Peace Is Every Step: The Path of Mindfulness in Everyday Life*. New York: Bantam, 1992.

Kabat-Zinn, Jon. *Wherever You Go, There You Are: Mindfulness Meditation in Everyday Life*. New York: Hyperion, 1994.

Keating, Thomas. *Open Mind, Open Heart: The Contemplative Dimension of the Gospel*. New York: Continuum, 1992.

Merton, Thomas. *Spiritual Direction and Meditation*. Collegeville, Minn.: The Liturgical Press, 1960.

Salzberg, Sharon. *Lovingkindness: The Revolutionary Art of Happiness*. Boston: Shambhala, 1997.

To learn more about meditation, please visit www.oneminutemeditator.com. The *One-Minute Meditator* Web site offers an inside look at the research behind the book. It also lists places to meditate with a teacher. Sign on and enjoy learning more about the meditation community on the Web.